The Critique of Regression

The Critique of Regression presents the most in-depth critique of regression available in the psychoanalytic literature, whilst presenting the first psychoanalytic theory of irreversible lifespan development. The clinical implications are amply demonstrated in three chapter-length psychoanalytic cases. The most important implication is that when we revisit the past, in a private memory or in an analytic session, we remake it afresh in light of the present. The analysis of the past is always, in this sense, an exploration of the present.

Gregory S. Rizzolo demonstrates that where we think we see returns, or regressions, to past stages of the lifespan, we in fact find the emergence of novel structures in subjective experience. Rizzolo considers the work of human development to be a work of mourning in which we lose, internalize and keep reworking the residue of a past to which we never return. The traditional notion of regression, which supports the fantasy of a literal return, operates as an intellectual defense against the mourning process. To critique the concept is to address the defense and to confront the loss of past relationships and of past versions of selfhood inherent in development. From the work of mourning emerge ever-new configurations of desire, defense and subjective meaning. The task of analysis is to cultivate, amidst the repetition of familiar patterns, the potential for novelty at play in each moment.

This thought-provoking work will interest new and experienced psychoanalytic clinicians alike, who want to go beyond traditional theories of development to a contemporary look at how we develop inexorably across the lifespan.

Gregory S. Rizzolo is a faculty member at the Institute for Clinical Social Work in Chicago and an advanced candidate at the Chicago Institute for Psychoanalysis. His work has appeared in *Psychoanalytic Psychology*, the *Psychoanalytic Study of the Child* and the *Journal of the American Psychoanalytic Association*. He maintains a private practice in Chicago USA.

When music is played in a new key, the melody does not change, but the notes that make up the composition do: change in the context of continuity, continuity that perseveres through change. Psychoanalysis in a New Key publishes books that share the aims psychoanalysts have always had, but that approach them differently. The books in the series are not expected to advance any particular theoretical agenda, although to this date most have been written by analysts from the Interpersonal and Relational orientations.

The most important contribution of a psychoanalytic book is the communication of something that nudges the reader's grasp of clinical theory and practice in an unexpected direction. Psychoanalysis in a New Key creates a deliberate focus on innovative and unsettling clinical thinking. Because that kind of thinking is encouraged by exploration of the sometimes surprising contributions to psychoanalysis of ideas and findings from other fields, Psychoanalysis in a New Key particularly encourages interdisciplinary studies. Books in the series have married psychoanalysis with dissociation, trauma theory, sociology, and criminology. The series is open to the consideration of studies examining the relationship between psychoanalysis and any other field—for instance, biology, literary and art criticism, philosophy, systems theory, anthropology, and political theory.

But innovation also takes place within the boundaries of psychoanalysis, and Psychoanalysis in a New Key therefore also presents work that reformulates thought and practice without leaving the precincts of the field. Books in the series focus, for example, on the significance of personal values in psychoanalytic practice, on the complex interrelationship between the analyst's clinical work and personal life, on the consequences for the clinical situation when patient and analyst are from different cultures, and on the need for psychoanalysts to accept the degree to which they knowingly satisfy their own wishes during treatment hours, often to the patient's detriment. A full list of all titles in this series is available at: https://www.routledge.com/series/LEAPNKBS

TITLES IN THIS SERIES INCLUDE:

Vol. 46 Travels with the Self
Interpreting Psychology as Cultural History
Philip Cushman

Vol. 45 The Critique of Regression
A Psychoanalytic Model of Irreversible Lifespan Development
Gregory S. Rizzolo

The Critique of Regression

A Psychoanalytic Model of Irreversible Lifespan Development

Gregory S. Rizzolo

Routledge
Taylor & Francis Group
LONDON AND NEW YORK

First published 2019
by Routledge
2 Park Square, Milton Park, Abingdon, Oxon OX14 4RN

and by Routledge
52 Vanderbilt Avenue, New York, NY 10017

Routledge is an imprint of the Taylor & Francis Group, an informa business

British Library Cataloguing-in-Publication Data
A catalogue record for this book is available from the British Library

Library of Congress Cataloging-in-Publication Data
Names: Rizzolo, Gregory S., author.
Title: The critique of regression : a psychoanalytic model of irreversible lifespan development / Gregory S. Rizzolo.
Description: Abingdon, Oxon ; New York, NY : Routledge, 2019. | Includes bibliographical references and index.
Identifiers: LCCN 2018014840 (print) | LCCN 2018017946 (ebook) | ISBN 9780429460876 (Master) | ISBN 9780429865022 (Web PDF) | ISBN 9780429865015 (ePub) | ISBN 9780429865008 (Mobipocket/Kindle) | ISBN 9781138624399 (hardback : alk. paper) | ISBN 9781138624405 (pbk. : alk. paper)
Subjects: LCSH: Regression (Psychology) | Psychoanalysis.
Classification: LCC RC489.R42 (ebook) | LCC RC489.R42 R59 2019 (print) | DDC 616.89/17—dc23
LC record available at https://lccn.loc.gov/2018014840

ISBN: 978-1-138-62439-9 (hbk)
ISBN: 978-1-138-62440-5 (pbk)
ISBN: 978-0-429-46087-6 (ebk)

Typeset in Times
by Apex CoVantage, LLC

For Mom & Dad
Doug & Trev
Grandma Cookie
Jess
&
Sienna Rose

Contents

Acknowledgments

Many people have helped me in developing these ideas and finding the words to express them. First and foremost, I would like to thank my mentor Karl Figlio, always ready to play the devil's advocate and yet equally encouraging of my independent thought, who has pushed me toward ever greater clarity in the argument I present in these pages. I also wish to thank, from the University of Essex, Matt Ffytche and Peter Dews, who shared their insight and offered much useful feedback on the manuscript over the years.

What I write is grounded in the clinical encounter. Without my patients, I would have little to theorize about. I therefore wish to give special thanks to my analysands, necessarily anonymous, who have inspired me, often, I suspect, in ways they do not realize.

A psychoanalytic clinician, ostensibly isolated in his office, never truly operates alone. I wish to thank David Terman, my first analytic supervisor at the Chicago Institute for Psychoanalysis, whose calm, warmth and intellect represent for me what is best about the field. I would also like to thank Mark Levey, who, in his patience, sensitivity and pragmatism, has become a model for me; Charles Jaffe, who taught me to track the micro-process of an analytic session; Michael Hoit, who modeled a warm and integrative ego psychology; and Robert Galatzer-Levy, open-minded almost to the point of chaos, who supervised the case of Travis in Chapter 10, and whose nonlinear approach to development provided the most immediate intellectual catalyst for my theory of the lifespan.

I might not have come to train at the Chicago Institute had not the director of the Adult Psychotherapy Clinic, Polly Everett, taken a chance in hiring me as a practicum student. I would like to thank Polly and the former directors of the student program, Kate Schechter and Jeff Seiden, for welcoming me in and introducing me to psychoanalytic practice. Beyond them, Don McDevitt and Dale Gody became indispensable early supervisors.

The Chicago Institute offers a one-year fellowship program for graduate students and early career professionals who want to get their feet wet. I would like to thank the director of the fellowship program, Caryle Perlman, who accepted me and paired me with my mentor Bonnie Litowitz. For a young and then unpublished writer, it was almost inconceivable to have the mentorship of such an accomplished scholar–clinician, one who would shortly become editor-in-chief at the *Journal of the American Psychoanalytic Association*. When I write, I still think back to the space and intellectual freedom I felt in her office.

The mark of a good journal submission process, in my view, is one in which the reviewers help the author to develop whatever might be the vaguely realized potential in his first draft. In this spirt, I would like to thank, in addition to Bonnie, Mitchell Wilson and the reviewers who critiqued my work at the *Journal of the American Psychoanalytic Association*. I would also like to thank Claudia Lament, Rona Knight and the reviewers at the *Psychoanalytic Study of the Child*. I am grateful to both journals for encouraging me to keep going and to produce stronger manuscripts than those that I originally sent them.

Apart from my patients, I have learned the most from my students and supervisees at the Institute for Clinical Social Work in Chicago. I am grateful to my colleagues and faculty mentors Scott Rose, Jennifer Tolleson, Woody Faigen, and Joan Servatius for giving me such great classes, and to my students and supervisees for their persistent questioning.

At Routledge, I would like to thank acquisitions editor Kate Hawes and series editor Donnel Stern, whose work I have admired since college, for taking a chance on a first-time author. Charles Bath has, in addition, been of great help in preparing the final manuscript.

Lastly, and most importantly for me, I would like to thank my wife Jess, a beautiful mother, a scholar of Animal Studies and a steadfast partner, who loves to point out the 'regressive' behavior we see and defies me playfully to say regression never happens.

Introduction

When we dream, Freud (1900) argued, we slip backwards from a world of conscious action into an unconscious realm of infantile memory and desire. The residues of our waking life meet there with repressed primitive wishes capable of animating a dream. "We may speak of dreams," he wrote, "as having a 'regressive' character" (p. 541).

The idea of regression, with all of its intrigue, would shape a century of theory building. It would also become one of the thorniest, if recently neglected, areas of inquiry.

The process of dreaming is, Freud (1900) continued, analogous to that of neurotic symptom formation (p. 597). A thought or behavior becomes pathological when it is seized upon and made into the disguised vehicle of expression for a repressed infantile wish. To unravel a symptom, as to unravel a dream, is to trace it back to its origin in infancy.

The libido theory articulated what Freud considered the most consequential of infantile wishes—the child's sexual impulses—and set them in a developmental series (Freud, 1905). The infant's pleasure in sucking at the breast gives rise, he held, to the oral phase; his pleasure in anal retention and elimination to the anal phase; and his phallic-genital interest in the opposite sex parent, and with it the Oedipus complex, to the phallic phase. A fixation in any phase could set the stage for a regressive neurosis in later life.

The articulation of theory led to a greater specificity in the kinds of regression it anticipated. In hysteria, for instance, it predicted a "regression of the libido to the primary incestuous sexual objects," that is to the Oedipus complex, but "no regression to an earlier stage of sexual organization" (Freud, 1917a, p. 342). The hysteric thus regards herself as the apple of her father's eye, but resents the impression, having noticed the little boy's penis, that she must accept a passive feminine position in the world (Freud, 1924).

In the obsessional neuroses, it anticipated, by contrast, a "regression of the libido to the preliminary stage of the sadistic-anal organization" (Freud, 1917a, p. 343). The obsessional thus evades the danger of castration by retreating into anal position from which vantage point he becomes preoccupied with control of dirty objects, feelings and impulses.

The history of psychoanalysis suggests a deepening interest in still earlier forms of regression. Zetzel (1968), for instance, introduced the "so-called good hysteric," a woman whose sexual interest in her father/analyst screens a pre-Oedipal fixation on her mother, who she feels deprived her of warmth and tenderness, much as the analyst now deprives her. The false self patient of Winnicott (1965) is more compliant than the so-called hysteric. He cooperates readily, but lifelessly, with the analysis of his Oedipus complex. Behind the compliance he too, however, betrays a deeper problem: a sense of non-existence masked by adaptation to maternal impingement now replicated in the analysis.

Balint's (1968) basic-fault patient and Kohut's (1971, 1977) narcissist belong to the same category of patients, who, though they might seem Oedipal, reveal, in their heightened vulnerability and/or deadened compliance, a variety of earlier regressive needs. The first person, who clings to others, or alternately learns skills to become self-sufficient, yearns unconsciously to return to the lost (or never realized) harmony of the mother–infant mix-up. The second, grandiose, but depressed and shame-prone, hungers for the mirroring, or the merger with an idealized other, that was thwarted in the earliest years.

The literature is peopled with character types dated to early childhood fixations and ruptures. The characters themselves are easy to find in everyday practice. The effort to provide an origin story for each one, leads, however, into two basic problems. First, it sets up hypotheses that cannot be verified beyond the tautological reconstruction of the adult's infancy. The impression is one of picking the wrong battles: The truth embodied in the character type, as a construct, is lost in unresolvable speculation about infantile causation. The stories tend, second, to be reductionist of life beyond childhood. The intrigue of later life can get lost in an aesthetic in which everything is contained in the beginning.

The first problem undermines efforts to address the second one. To address the second problem, one might take a three-step approach: (a) verify the theory's picture of childhood, (b) verify the theory's picture of the adult's neurosis, and (c) demonstrate an empirical correlation the strength of which shows that later development is redundant or irrelevant. The difficulty, however, which brings us back to the first problem, is that the picture of childhood typically refers to motives and phantasies that lie beyond empirical verification. It would seem that the picture of childhood can be modified at whim to perfect the correlation until we are left with a restatement of the adult in the image of the baby.

We find scattered attempts to approach this tangle. Hartmann (1955) cautions against the 'genetic fallacy' whereby we reduce present-day mentation to its infantile precursors as if the continuity of function were inconsistent the development of function. Erikson (1958) similarly pokes fun at what he calls "originology": "a habit of thinking which reduces every human situation to an analogy with an earlier one, and most of all to that earliest, simplest and most infantile precursor which is assumed to be its 'origin'" (p. 18).

The theoretical swerve to originology has garnered too little interest. It is unlikely that anyone would appeal, for the sake of comparison, to the theory of the primal horde (Freud, 1913b) to explain contemporary social phenomena like the rise of ISIS, Brexit or the election of Trump. It is evident, regardless of the validity or invalidity of such origin myths, that one would require a more contemporary history of the issues or movements in question. Why do we accept a similar kind of lacunae, then, in our explanation of adult disorders?

Mitchell (1988) argued that the field of psychoanalysis holds to a latent morality of maturity by which it locates the most uncomfortable aspects of human experience in the child. The readiness to originology might reflect a moral impulse, then, to infantilize the patient. The analyst and often the patient tacitly accept the idea that the most unruly impulses, needs, affects, defenses and phantasies in human experience are, by definition, childish. The psyche is split accordingly into the mature and the infantile. The patient and analyst join in the belief that, of the two of them, the patient is the more immature one.

The theoretically sanctioned move to infantilize the patient might serve a number of purposes. It might make the patient's provocative or emotional nature more acceptable and even endearing. It is often easier to forgive in a 'child' what would be unacceptable in an adult. It might, at the same time, afford the analyst a momentary feeling of triumph over the 'childish' parts of himself that he has unconsciously identified with his childish patient.

The implication is that the theory of regression can provide an intellectual safe-haven for unanalyzed countertransference feelings toward the so-called childish parts of the patient. To challenge the theory is, therefore, to open an unwelcome area of analytic inquiry.

The inquiry itself leads into the network of beliefs, concepts and images that give rise to the problem. Freud (1937) pictured the mind as an archeological dig site. The relics of infantile sexuality were thought to be buried beneath the corroding effects of everyday weather. The causal hypothesis is that the infantile persists because it is repressed and, as such, can surge up to influence, but is not much altered by, events in the present. Such a vision supports the possibility of a regression to unmodified infantile fixations.

Wachtel (2003) points out, however, that early patterns drop out of the lifespan if they are not reinforced. A different causal hypothesis emerges. The infantile persists, to the extent that it does, not because it is buried beneath present influences, but because it is inextricably implicated in shaping the present and is continually reinforced by its own effects.

To concede this point, but retain the concept of regression, one might invoke the imagery of ego psychology. The ego, then, is a machine comprised of functions and sub-functions (Hartmann, Kris, & Loewenstein, 1946). The best functions are mature and durable. Other functions are less so. They can break down and regress to earlier modes of operation (Arlow & Brenner, 1964). Production continues, in that event, on the basis of a compromise between the stable-mature and the regressed functions of the operating system.

The problem here is one of the genetic fallacy. It is assumed that the structural continuity from a past ego function to a present one is inconsistent with the notion of development. Certainly, one can reify a given mental function—a supposedly regressed function in this case—and then artificially isolate the parts that best show its childhood origins. The function is not a thing, however, but a way of operating. It has become part and parcel of a broader personality style. It is integrated with other functions, in the service of new interests and demands, such that its functional status is not what it was in childhood.

I shall argue that, contrary to the theory of regression, the person develops irreversibly across the lifespan. The work of development is, in large part, a work of mourning in which we lose, internalize and keep reworking the residues of a past to which we never return. The psychoanalytic notion of regression, which supports the fantasy of a literal return, operates, even behind any morality of maturity, as a defense against the loss inherent in development. We can more accurately describe what we once called 'regressions' as shifts, or transformations, in the present intrapsychic–interpersonal field. The personality styles above, so eloquently described by their authors, are best seen as lifespan adaptations. No one makes a pure return to the subjective world of his infancy.[1]

The book is organized into ten chapters in which I trace the history of the concept of regression, discuss past and present critiques, and attempt to substantiate the argument above.

The first chapter presents what I have termed the traditions of defensive and restorative regression (Rizzolo, 2016). The defensive tradition frames regression as a retreat from the dangers of forward development. The restorative tradition frames regression, by contrast, as a primary (non-defensive) pull toward a restorative object relationship. I discuss the first tradition, which originates in Freud, the second tradition, which originates in Ferenczi, and integrationists, like Balint, Winnicott and Kohut, who constructed developmental tilt models (Mitchell, 1988) in order to house both potential regressions.

The second chapter examines earlier conservative and radical critiques of the concept. The conservative critique holds that the term is misused and/or misapplied in clinical practice (Macalpine, 1950; Arlow & Brenner, 1964; Gill, 1984a). The implication is that it should be revised or clarified. The radical critique suggests that the term—no matter how well it is clarified—leads to the genetic fallacy and, behind it, a morality of maturity (Mitchell, 1988; Inderbitzin & Levy, 2000; Rizzolo, 2016). The implication is that it should be abandoned in favor of a more nuanced sense of the infusion of past and present.

The third chapter, which attempts to develop the implications of the radical critique, argues that the person—an irreducible agent of his own experience—is the proper subject of psychoanalytic inquiry (Schafer, 1976; Gill, 1983; Stolorow, Brandchaft, & Atwood, 1987). The person thinks, feels and acts out of the whole of his inner composition. It does not make sense, then, to parse the doings of his repressed infantile self from those of his adult self. Nor does it make sense to parse the workings of infantile functions from later ones. The early and later acquired functions merge into the present movement.

The fourth chapter explores the relational matrix in which the person makes meaning of his experience. Traditional psychoanalytic conceptualizations argued for the regressive nature of group functioning (Freud, 1921; Bion, 1961). A related but distinct wave of pre-Oedipal theorizing emphasized the infantile nature of intense interpersonal dependency (Hartmann, 1939; Winnicott, 1954a, 1954b; Balint, 1968; Mahler, 1975; Kohut, 1971). A tautology emerges in which it is presupposed that only children are intensely dependent on others; intense dependency in later life thus becomes evidence of regression. But it is by now a commonplace that we are all embedded in fields of dependency. The tautology is rejected for a broader conception of *Nachträglichkeit* (Freud, 1896, 1898, 1918), or deferred action, in which the past is continuously reshaped in the field of our present dependencies. Our ongoing dependency becomes, therefore, not the evidence of regression, but rather a precondition in re-imagining the past.

I illustrate the deferred action of the field through Klein's (1959) apt portrayal of how marriage changes the psyche in depth. We observe in her account how the wife reconfigures her husband's internal mother and, conversely, how he reconfigures her internal father. The changes exemplify how the present field in fact modifies all internal figures.

I proceed to a special case of deferred action in the adult representation of child selves. The imagined figure, or character, is not the direct portrait of an historical self, but a construction—expressive a lifespan history—configured or reconfigured in the present field. I illustrate this point in Davies and Frawley's (1991) vivid account of the child representation one often finds in the internal world of adult survivors of childhood sexual abuse.

The fifth chapter attempts to bring the person and the field into a lifespan model of development.[2] The unconscious is considered 'timeless,' or lacking in temporal distinctions. Yet it is nested in a lifespan history and so, contrary to Freud's view, reflects the inexorable passage of time. The person must therefore face the constant loss a past to which he cannot return. Instead of dating common clinical issues, for example trust, autonomy and assertiveness, to nodal infantile fixations or arrests, I reframe them as issues for the life cycle (Stern, 1985; Mitchell, 1988). The person does not regress to them, but reengages them in new iterations at each new phase of life (Wachtel, 2003, 2008). The entry into each new phase opens new fields with unique limits and growth potentials. The struggle is rarely uniform.

For most people, it involves shifts between modes (Erikson, 1950) and positions (Klein, 1946; Waddell, 1998) within the relational matrix.

No one can roll back the additions and modifications of lifespan development in a full-fledged return to the motives and conflicts of his childhood. By *regression*, however, some analysts mean not a full-fledged return to an earlier developmental phase, but a non-phase-specific slip into primitive phantasies and defenses. The operational term, in this particular variation, is not regression, but *primitive*, which originated in Freud's (1913b) interest in anthropology. Freud and his followers, including Klein, believed in a world where ontogeny recapitulates phylogeny. Here the regressed analysand = normative child = third-world subject = primitive subject. The sixth chapter queries the basic assumption that primitive psychology is, in fact, primitive.[3] I argue, in the negative, that many so-called primitive processes—for example, hallucinatory gratification, condensation, splitting and projective identification—are not intrinsically primary in evolution or development. They develop from infantile to adult modes of operation. To engage in them is not to regress, but to make use of increasingly sophisticated mental operations.

The seventh chapter addresses the relatively recent psychoanalytic interest in the here-and-now. The relational, Kleinian and ego-psychological theorists of the here-and-now share an interest, in spite of their metapsychological differences, in the analysis of transference, and, except for Gill, in the analysis of present extra-analytic manifestations of conflict (Joseph, 1978, 1989, 2013; Gill, 1979, 1984b; Sandler & Sandler, 1984, 1987, 1994a). For them the analysis of the present comes before and takes priority over genetic interpretation. The critique of regression clarifies that the analysis of the here-and-now is not a superficial activity, that is, a game played with the derivatives of buried infantile mentation, but, on the contrary, an engagement at the deepest levels of the present unconscious. The reconstruction of infancy is not an inherently profound activity, but rather a narrative act, which reflects, in form and content, the subject's immersion in the field.

The eighth chapter explores the clinical implications in a contemporary report of defensive regression (Haft, 2005). A hermeneutic methodology is advanced to suit the purpose. It aims not to disprove what cannot be disproven—namely, claims about the repressed infantile past—but to move beyond genetic reconstruction to a more complete lifespan conceptualization. The patient, then, who presents with severe obsessive-compulsive symptoms, is thought by the analyst to have regressed from Oedipal dangers to an anal fixation. The symptoms emerge, it is held, to manage anal erotic and sadistic impulses. I attempt to show that, regardless of potential anal influences, we require a lifespan conceptualization. The patient experiences his erotic-sadistic impulses through an ever-evolving identification with his father—one that proceeds through several life phase iterations. We can understand the image of the anal toddler not as a literal picture of the patient's unconscious self, but as a character with meaning in the here-and-now field.

The ninth chapter pursues the implications further in a contemporary report of restorative regression (Grossmark, 2012). The patient, who feels he does not exist, relies on a war chest of erotic and sadistic behaviors to ward off a profound and empty sense of despair. He can be aloof, insightful, needy, rejecting, appreciative, desperately excited and so on. The analyst is forbidden, however, to interpret his mood or even to request that he attend his sessions, rather, than, say, calling in impromptu from the car or the shower. The analyst suggests that the patient has regressed to a primary state of mother–infant relating. The difficult behavior, it is thought, reflect an infantile demand for total attunement. I attempt to demonstrate, by contrast, that the behavior, like the obsessional symptoms in the previous chapter, require a lifespan interpretation. It reflects an erotized identification with a dominant mother rolled into a sadistic identification with an abusive step-father and subsequently cultivated through the actual domination of men in fetish clubs. The image of the patient as a neonate appears in the relational matrix. It helps the analyst to endure the patient's needy demands and softens his guilty countertransference frustration.

The tenth chapter presents a lifespan approach to the analysis of a young man, a thwarted singer-songwriter, who sought help for jealous thoughts he felt undermined his reality-testing.[4] Travis worried that his lovers, of whom there were several, merely tolerated him. They lusted, in secret, after his more aggressive and successful rivals—or so he believed. I provide a developmental history and three representative sessions. I then suggest how a defensive and restorative regression analyst might conceptualize the process. The two regression accounts illuminate relevant childhood dynamics. But they leave open three gaps. They do not, for one, account for the specificity at play in the associations. Travis finds himself in rivalry with a specific male object (the rival artist) for a specific female object (the feminine muse). They reflect his childhood parents only through the later prism of his adolescent/young adult search for an identity in artistic production. They do not account, second, for the fear he has grounded his worth in a grandiose illusion. They do not touch, lastly, on the mourning implicit in accepting that he has failed to actualize his teenage dreams and in moving forward toward a revised vision. A lifespan interpretation accounts for these gaps. It brings the childhood insights of the first two accounts into a further reaching analysis of the tasks and dangers in the present.

My primary aim in this book is to explore a vision of psychoanalysis without regression. To abandon the term is to resist the genetic fallacy and the often implicit morality of maturity. It is, moreover, to confront the loss inherent in irreversible lifespan development. It is not, however, to dismiss the character types embedded in regression theory. The causality is simply redistributed from childhood, which we have over-privileged, to a cumulative causality of reinforcements and modifications in each phase of life. The field of inquiry is opened, by implication, into the function of patient-infantilization and, beyond this point, into the often subtle transformations of lifelong development.

Notes

1 An earlier version of this critique appeared in the *Journal of the American Psychoanalytic Association*, 64(6): 1097–1131.
2 An earlier version of this chapter has been accepted for publication in *The Psychoanalytic Study of the Child* (Rizzolo, in press).
3 An earlier version of this chapter appeared in the *Journal of the American Psychoanalytic Association* 65(6): 945–977.
4 A shorter version of this case has been accepted for publication in *The Psychoanalytic Study of the Child.*

Chapter 1

The Defensive and Restorative Traditions

The term *regression* has been used in many different ways since Freud's early (1900) discussion of the formal, temporal and topographical aspects of regression in dreaming. Two dominant traditions—here termed the 'defensive' and 'restorative' traditions—have evolved, along with several integrative traditions, in the psychoanalytic literature.

The individual retreats, in a defensive regression, from a situation of unconscious danger to an earlier fixation of relative safety and pleasure. He replaces current wishes and dangers with the more manageable, if still problematic, ones from an earlier phase of life. The process of regression is likened metaphorically to the flow of a stream that washes back on itself (Freud, 1905) or to the retreat of an army to an old camp (Freud, 1917a).

In a restorative regression, by contrast, the subject experiences a primary yearning to re-establish early conditions of merger with a life-sustaining other who is felt to be an environment. This is not a defensive process. It is mobilized by feelings of safety, not of danger. Such regressions can be likened metaphorically to a merger with Thalassa, the primal sea spirit (Ferenczi, 1938), a harmonious mix-up in the mother–infant dyad (Balint, 1968), or the inhale of the other's pride and joy as a kind of oxygen (Kohut, 1984).

In Balint, Winnicott and Kohut's writing we find similar attempts to integrate the defensive and restorative regression traditions into a comprehensive model of mental functioning. They rely, in spite of their differences, on a common 'developmental tilt' approach (Mitchell, 1988). Dependency needs are located in the pre-Oedipal years of development. Restorative regressions are thus thought to imply a return to pre-Oedipal needs. Sexual and aggressive conflicts, and retreats from them, are considered Oedipal in nature. Defensive regressions are thus thought to imply a higher level of developmental achievement.

In spite of its explanatory appeal, however, the developmental tilt highlights problems internal to the concept of regression. Above all, it raises the problem of the genetic fallacy (Hartmann, 1955). We find ubiquitous relational needs reduced to their original manifestations in early life in spite of widespread clinical findings that such needs are pervasive among so-called pre-Oedipal and Oedipal patients across the life cycle. The reduction suggests an implicit a morality of maturity vis-à-vis dependency needs. The internal break down of this solution re-opens an inquiry into the problems of regression.

The Tradition of Defensive Regression

The psychoanalytic concept of regression first appears in Freud's *Interpretation of Dreams* (1900). "We call it 'regression,'" he wrote, "when in a dream an idea is turned back into the sensory image from which it was originally derived" (p. 543). According to the theory, the process integrates three different kinds of regression. There is a 'formal' regression from complex ideas to primitive sensory images, a 'topographical' regression from the preconscious to the conscious systems, and a 'temporal' regression from present to past psychic structures. The three kinds of regression were held to be 'one at bottom,' because, "what is older in time is more primitive in form and in psychical topography lies nearer to the perceptual end" (p. 548).

Freud developed the concept further in his *Three Essays on the Theory of Sexuality* (1905). Here he introduces a psychic force—the libido—that can progress or regress along an organically determined line of development. The libido is defined as a quantitative variable representing 'processes' and 'transformations' in sexual excitation (p. 83). It flows from a narcissistic reservoir of self-cathexis into oral, anal and genital object investments. Along the way, it forms fixation points of relative safety and gratification. If it encounters obstacles—for example, danger situations—in its forward path, it can regress, washing back like a blocked 'stream,' into the 'channels' of its old fixations (p. 170).

He later suggested that the ego marches in step with the libido (Freud, 1916–1917). If the libido behaves like a stream, the ego behaves like an army. It establishes camps along the path of libidinal development to which it can retreat, as needed, from conflict on the front line.

The concept of regression became an essential diagnostic tool. In hysteria, for example, there was thought to be a regression to the "primary incestuous objects" of the OedipalOedipal phase (Freud, 1916–1917, p. 342). In the obsessional neuroses, by contrast, there was held to be a deeper regression from Oedipal danger to an anal-sadistic fixation wherein the libidinal impulse was "obliged . . . to disguise itself as a sadistic impulsion" (pp. 343–344). Paranoia, in this theory, reflected an even deeper regression from object love to narcissism. It left a dry riverbed of object libido—not enough to form a transference to the analysts—rendering the patient inaccessible by the psychoanalytic method (Freud, 1912, 1914).

Ego psychology expanded in various ways upon the work of regression in human development. We find, for instance, normal and pathological regressions along the developmental lines of id, ego and superego (A. Freud, 1965), progressive and regressive ego adaptations (Hartman, 1939), regression in psychic differentiation and integration (Hartmann, Kris, & Loewenstein, 1946), regression in the service of the ego (Kris, 1936) and, more recently, the anti-regressive function of the ego (Sandler & Sandler, 1994b).

'Psychoanalysis,' Gill (1954) wrote, in a statement that, for many, captured the essence of clinical practice, "is that technique which, employed by a neutral analyst, results in the development of a regressive transference neurosis and the ultimate resolution of this neurosis by techniques of interpretation alone" (p. 775). Implicitly excluded from analysis were those patients considered to be too regressed to tolerate the analyst's neutrality or, in the most withdrawn and psychotic cases, to form a neurotic transference.

At the same time, we also find in ego psychology a certain complication of the concept of regression: Its potential adaptive-progressive value emerges, such that the concept no longer refers so clearly to a return to the past. Hartmann (1939) wrote, for instance, that even when mature forms of mentation fail, and a regressive adaptation presents itself to fill the gap, "no pure form of a previous developmental stage emerges" (p. 50). The regressive mentation has, paradoxically, a novel quality in the present. It is a solution to a new problem and, in its novelty of function, becomes part of new psychic structure.

Loewald (1981) seemed to acknowledge the latent conceptual problems when he wrote that, "words and concepts (such as regression and the rest) reveal themselves as flimsy or enigmatic or ambiguous if they are not merely used as shortcuts and as currency in the exchange of thoughts but are given weight and consideration in their own right" (p. 22). He argued in favor of retaining the concept as a shortcut. One might counter-argue, however, that it is by exploring latent conceptual flimsiness that space opens for new thought.

Although Melanie Klein departed from the ego psychological reading of Freud, she too framed regression as a defensive retreat from situations of internal conflict and danger. In her writing, however, the standard picture of regression is complicated by regressive-progressive oscillation between the paranoid-schizoid and depressive positions:

> For if persecutory fear, and correspondingly schizoid mechanisms, are too strong, the ego is not capable of working through to the depressive position. This forces the ego to regress to the paranoid-schizoid position and reinforces earlier persecutory fears and schizoid phenomena.
> [Klein, 1946, p. 15]

The oscillation between positions is not phase specific. It can occur within any phase of life. It does not, that is, imply an erotogenic regression. This complicates the picture. It arguably opens the door for a re-imagining of regressions as shifts that occur within phases of the life cycle. I pursue this direction in Chapters 4 and 5.

Klein also implicitly challenged the concept of regression in her contention that the Oedipus complex manifests in oral phase of the first year of life (Klein, 1928, 1945). "The frustration experienced at the mother's breast," she wrote, "leads both boy and girl to turn away from it and stimulates the infant's desire for oral gratification from the penis of the father" (Klein, 1945, p. 408). It is a matter of controversy whether the infant has the mental capacity to form a phantasy of the father's penis. Whether or not Klein's assertion is correct, it suggests that the Oedipal situation is not bounded within the confines of the phallic-genital phase, but, on the contrary, can occur in so-called pre-Oedipal phases. It is, in essence, an issue of triangular love relations that can occur in any phase.

Britton (1992) explores this opening in his contention that the Oedipal situation is 'never finished,' but has to be "re-worked in each new life situation, at each stage of development, and with each major addition to experience or knowledge" (p. 38). We do not regress to the Oedipal situation; we rework it over and over again.

The Tradition of Restorative Regression

In 1914, Ferenczi attempted an interpretation and elaboration of Freud's libido theory. Ferenczi's reading, published in 1938 under the title *Thalassa,* indulged in what he admitted to be a loose, but arguably fruitful, play with mythical and biological metaphors. He argued that libidinal striving expresses a universal longing to return an 'aquatic' mode of existence, which the infant first experienced in the womb, and which was first experienced by proto-organisms in the ocean. There is a trace of the sea in the womb, so to speak, and one is always trying to get back to the state of repose experienced there. "The human being is dominated," he wrote, "from the moment of birth onwards by a continuous regressive trend toward the reestablishment of the intrauterine situation" (p. 20).

For Freud and the ego psychologists, psychosexual development followed a path from primary narcissism to differentiation and ultimately genital investment in a separate object. Ferenczi held, by contrast, that genitality was not an achievement of the differentiated ego, but, on the contrary, the expression of a deep regressive longing for merger. "The purpose . . . of the sex act . . . can be none other than an attempt on the part of the ego . . . to return to the mother's womb, where there is no . . . painful disharmony between ego and environment" (p. 18).

Just as Freud appealed to the metaphor of the stream in formulating the libido theory, Ferenczi appealed to the metaphor of Thalassa, the primeval sea spirit who spawned the first life forms. The mother's body symbolizes the primeval ocean from which life emerged, and to which it longs to return—to a state of harmony prior to the trauma of separation. The libido is not just pleasure seeking, then, but also Thalassa-seeking.

Balint (1959, 1968) acknowledges the influence of Ferenczi's *Thalassa* more than any other theorist in the restorative regression tradition. He draws explicitly on the metaphor of Thalassa in his depiction of the mother–infant dyad:

> The child safely held in its mother's arms, the intrauterine, and the thalassal existence—are to be considered as symbolically identical; the friendly expanses of my theory are then but wish-fulfilling memories of these states; conversely, these states activate a strong attraction for regression.
>
> (1959, p. 96)

'Basic fault' patients, that is those who suffered early traumas of mis-satunement in the mother–infant dyad, require a restorative regression to the thalassal harmony of primary love:

> The patient must be allowed to regress . . . to the particular form of object relationship which caused the original deficiency state. Only after that can the patient "begin anew," that is, develop new patterns of object relationship.
>
> (pp. 165–166)

As for the analyst, he

> must do everything in his power not to become, or to behave as, a separate, sharply countered object. In other words, he must allow his patients to relate to, or exist with, him as if he were one of the primary substances. This means he should be willing to carry the patient, not actively, but like water carries the swimmer . . . that is, to be used without too much resistance against being used.
>
> (p. 167)

The regression here is not a defensive retreat. To interpret it as such would, in fact, constitute a resistance, on the analyst's part, to the terror of self-loss in a merger with the patient. It must be recognized and met as a primary striving to facilitate the patient's growth.

Winnicott and Kohut avoid any such explicit link to Ferenczi's *Thalassa*. Kohut (1959), in fact, dismissed it for its speculative, non-psychoanalytic character. One can, nonetheless, discern a congruent theoretical trend in their conceptualization of restorative regression.

Winnicott (1954a, 1954b, 1955) described primary regression, for instance, in the analysis of borderlines, to a state of dependency in which the analyst becomes a good-enough mother in a holding environment. "In so far as the patient is regressed," he wrote, "the couch *is* the analyst, the pillows *are* breasts, the analyst *is* the mother at a certain past era" (italics in original) (1954a, p. 288). The analyst–mother's provision constitutes a holding environment in which spontaneous gestures of omnipotence, destruction and play can emerge and be survived without too much impingement or retaliation. The relaxation of false self-structures—the legacy of impingement in the original mother–infant dyad—allows for the emergence of a more vigorous and authentic self.

Kohut (1971, 1977, 1984) argued, along similar but different lines, for the remobilization and working through of regressive selfobject strivings in the analytic relationship. As the term, a selfobject striving involves a merger between oneself and the object. The merger is not a retreat from differentiation, but a source of nourishment and growth. In the most archaic expression of the mirror transference, for example, "the analyst is experienced as an extension of the grandiose self and he is referred to only insofar as he has become the carrier of the grandiosity and exhibitionism of the analysand's grandiose self" (1971, p. 114). There is a diffusion of boundaries such that the analyst's unobtrusive and affirming responsiveness become part of the patient's self-structure.

Where Ferenczi and Balint drew on oceanic imagery, and Winnicott on the imagery of the mother's lap, Kohut (1984) enlists the environmental imagery of oxygen. "A move from dependence (symbiosis) to independence (autonomy) in the psychological sphere is no more possible, let alone desirable," he wrote, "than a corresponding move from a life dependent on oxygen to a life independent of it in the biological sphere" (p. 47). In the revival of thwarted regressive selfobject strivings, the analyst becomes like the air—not a separate object—but a vital substance absorbed into the patient's self-structure.

The Developmental Tilt

The defensive and restorative regression traditions fit together—awkwardly—in what Mitchell (1988) called the 'developmental tilt' solution. A diagnostic response, it attempts to differentiate between the supposedly more infantile disorders of relational trauma, deficit and arrest (e.g., borderline, schizoid and narcissistic personalities) and the allegedly more mature disorders of conflict (e.g., hysteria and obsessional neuroses). It suggests that relational needs are primary in infancy and drive conflicts central in later childhood. Early formed relational defenses/adaptations become the uneven ground, in Mitchell's metaphor. Upon this uneven ground are built the leaning toward drive conflict.

Balint, Winnicott and Kohut present different variants on the developmental tilt solution. The classical hysteric and obsessional neurotic (see Freud, 1916–1917, pp. 342–423) remain, for each of them, the prime examples of the relatively well structured conflict disorders. The 'basic fault' disorders (Balint, 1968), the narcissistic personality and behavior disorders (Kohut, 1971; Kohut & Wolf, 1978), and the borderline patient

(Winnicott, 1965) become, in different ways, privileged examples of the early deficit disorders.

The earlier disorders are thought to reflect relational trauma in the parent–child dyad and are therefore believed to necessitate a restorative regression in the analytic setting. The aim is to provide an unobtrusive environment in which development can resume. The higher disorders are thought to reflect greater structuralization. The patient has achieved a relatively stable, differentiated ego. He relates to his objects as separate objects. Typically, he has entered into an Oedipal conflict and stayed there or regressed defensively. To work with this more sophisticated patient, one must establish a therapeutic alliance (Zetzel, 1956; Greenson, 1965), that is, a collaborative identification between the patient's observing ego and the analyst's analytic function (Sterba, 1934). It is not the primary vehicle of therapeutic action; rather, like the unobjectionable positive transference (Freud, 1912), of which it is the theoretical heir, it is a prerequisite for the successful analysis of motive, conflict and defense. The aim here is ego expansion and integration.

In his later writing, Kohut (1977, 1984) questioned the validity of this diagnostic approach. As we have already seen, he abandoned the idea that merger was an early phenomenon in favor of the view that selfobject fusion is essential to human existence across the life cycle. The child does not, therefore, grow out of narcissistic selfobject strivings into Oedipal drives and conflicts. Rather, the Oedipus complex becomes, in the revision of his original formulation, another phase of selfobject relating. In this phase, the child seeks a prideful affirmation from the rival parent of his or her budding competitiveness, on the one hand, and on the other hand, from the desired parent of his or her male or female attractiveness (Kohut, 1977; Terman, 1984). The parents' joyful acceptance (or rejection, seduction, exploitation etc.) becomes part of the child's self-structure.

The self-psychological position is reminiscent of Ferenczi's (1938) contention that genital striving aimed not for a differentiated pleasure but for a kind of harmonious merger. Already this claim had problematized the notion that one grows out of merger needs.

Mitchell (1988), who pushed this trend further, argued that psychological reality operates within 'relational matrix' that "encompasses both intrapsychic and interpersonal realms" (p. 9). Across the life cycle, human beings seek different forms of connection, security, dependency, merger, pleasure, mutuality etc. It follows that one cannot house relational needs within the pre-Oedipal years or, by extension, within the diagnostic population of borderlines and/or narcissists. A diagnostic solution is inappropriate to an ontological claim: that we are all interdependent, at the deepest levels, not just in infancy, but for life.

The researcher can always find, by implication, earlier versions of later relational issues, for example, fusion and separation, and claim for them a linear causal significance. It can appear that the present issue is merely the expression of a regressive issue preserved in the depths of the mind. But such a logic discounts the possibility of qualitative developmental differences between the past and the present. It also neglects more recent historical and contemporary causal factors that might shape and reinforce the new version.

There is, finally, an implicit morality of maturity (Mitchell, 1988) in the classical view of the analyst as a reasonable adult and the analysand as a needy or petulant child in the room. If the motives and feeling states in question are not uniquely childish, but simply human, then it seems doubly defensive (a) to disavow and project them into the image of the 'child' and (b) to proceed as if the analysand were the embodiment of this construct.

Two problems emerge, then, for the theory of regression. The first is that of the genetic fallacy (Hartmann, 1955): the potential reduction of psychological processes and phenomena, for example, merger phenomena, to their original manifestations, for example, in earliest infancy. The second is that of countertransference morality. What if the genetic fallacy is motivated? What purpose/s might it serve, for example, to imagine the patient as a child—as small, as less responsible, as perhaps easier to love, or as easier to forgive? To question the concept of regression is not just to explore and potentially revise one's theory of development, but also to consider, nested within it, the analyst's motives and purposes.

Chapter 2

The Conservative and Radical Critiques

To approach the critique of regression is itself to enter into a long psychoanalytic tradition. A number of conservative and radical critiques of regression have appeared over time. The conservative critics call out the lack of clarity in the term and/or its misuses in clinical practice (Macalpine, 1950; Arlow & Brenner, 1964; Gill, 1984a). The implication is that the term should be clarified and better regulated in its clinical application.

The proponents of a more radical revision suggest, by contrast, that the essential problem lies not in a lack of clarity or clinical misapplication, but in an implicit morality of maturity (Mitchell, 1988) that perpetuates a genetic fallacy (Hartmann, 1955) in our thinking. The solution, here, is not to revise the concept, but to replace it with a model of shifts, or transformations, with no claim of return to the unmodified phenomena of earlier times.

The conservative approach relies on traditional vision of depth in the dynamic unconscious. The deep unconscious is thought to preserve unmodified relics of infantile life. The person can regress unconsciously to the relics beneath the surface of his adult adaptations. The metaphor of depth depends, however, on the problematic assumption that the infantile persists unmodified because it is repressed and so buffered against later influence. This prejudice hinders our recognition of the way in which later development does, in fact, impact infantile patterns, reinforcing, updating and modifying them over time.

To save the concept of regression, one might appeal to the ego psychological metaphor of the mind-as-machine. The mind is then seen as a machine that we can break down into stable/mature and unstable/regression-prone functions. The machine itself is always a product of the present. But it relies on the coordination of mature and regressed operations. The metaphor of the machine reveals, however, an inevitable tendency to anthropomorphize the functions in question. The anthropomorphization of functions suggests that, behind this artificial view, there is an indivisible person who pulls the levers. It would seem that all activities of the person are inextricably embedded in the present.

The conceptual problems of the conservative critique reveal the untenable nature of a revised regression theory. The stage is set, then, to develop and flesh out a stronger critique.

The Conservative Critique

There is a history of criticism in psychoanalysis around the concept of regression. The critiques fall broadly into a conservative camp, which retains and attempts to clarify the concept, and a radical camp, which rejects the concept in favor of a model of irreversible lifespan development.

Macalpine (1950) argued, in perhaps the earliest critique of the concept, that analytic technique—for example, the use of the couch, the constancy of the environment, diminished personal responsibility in sessions, the full sympathetic attention of another being, and the frustration of gratification—creates an infantile setting to which the analysand must adapt by regression. Her argument went against the conventional view that the analytic situation mobilizes a spontaneous regression in the analysand. "It can no longer be maintained," she wrote, "that the analysand's reactions in analysis occur spontaneously. His behavior is a response to the rigid infantile setting to which he is exposed" (p. 525).

The critical direction of Macalpine's thought did not lead her to question the technical utility of regression. She argued, instead, for a theoretical recognition of the analyst's deliberate role in inducing regression for therapeutic purposes. She suggested that, in the first stage of analysis, the analysand must adapt to the infantile setting. In the second stage, his regression is established. Here, "the analysand represents the infant at various stages of development." The analyst continues to frustrate his wishes and thereby propel a further regression: "Under constant pressure of analytic frustration, he withdraws progressively to earlier, 'safer' infantile patterns of behavior, and the level of his conflict is sooner or later reached." The third, or terminal, stage of analysis consists, finally, of a "gradual retracing of the way back into adulthood towards a newly won independence" (p. 528).

In their later revision of psychoanalytic metapsychology, Arlow and Brenner (1964) argued that regression is not a 'global process,' involving the entire psychic apparatus, but rather a discrete process impacting only certain parts and functions of the structure (p. 63). One should not assume, for the sake of illustration, that just "because depressions are based upon a regression to an oral instinctual fixation point . . . the patient [is] returning to the oral phase of existence; in other words, that he [is becoming] a helpless infant once again, experiencing all objects as breast or mother, and pursuing exclusively passive, dependent patterns of activity in all aspects of his life." One should consider, by contrast, how certain functions have regressed to the oral phase, while others have not.

Arlow and Brenner further addressed what they considered a common false inference that, "derivatives of a particular instinctual wish must have originated during the phase in the individual's history when the drive from which that wish derived was dominant in mental life" (p. 64). One might assume, for instance, that an oral wish originated in the oral phase. But the "cannibalistic wish to devour the father . . . acquire his prowess, become like him, and take his place, is," they assert, "a typical wish of the Oedipus phase." One must consider not just the manifest content of the wish, which might correlate superficially with one or another phase, but also, and more importantly, the latent content. The latter might reveal needs, wishes and defenses from a different phase entirely.

They proposed that a clarification of terms would help analysts to avoid these and other similar mistakes. They clarified the term regression to mean: "the *re-emergence* [italics in original] of modes of mental functioning which were characteristic of the psychic activity of the individual during earlier periods of development" (p. 71). They intended their definition to encompass a 'primitivization' in functioning in any part of the mental apparatus: id drives, ego defenses and adaptations, and superego functions and trends.

With this definition in mind, they proceed to outline four essential features of the term:

1. "Regression is a universal tendency of mental functioning" (p. 72). This means that "the level of operation of any mental function is subject to *continuous flux* [italics mine] reflecting the revival of primitive wishes or reactivating modes of functioning which were characteristic for the individual during the early years of his life."

2. "Primitive forms of mental activity are persistent and may exist side by side with more mature forms of mental functioning" (p. 73).
3. "Regression is not necessarily permanent" (p. 74). Most regressions are 'temporary' and 'reversible.'
4. "As a rule regressions are specific and discrete in nature rather than global and total" (p. 75). There is often some interplay between regressive and non-regressive mentation.

Gill (1984a) went further than either Macalpine or Arlow and Brenner in his critique of regression. In an earlier paper of 1954, he had maintained that psychoanalytic technique results, if competently applied, in the development of a regressive transference neurosis (see Chapter 1). In a shift of perspective, he now discarded as illusory the very notion that the psychoanalytic process is capable of reinstating an earlier state in the patient:

> The argument that regression is a necessary part of the analytic method is based on the idea that an earlier infantile neurosis has to be revived and resolved. I believe that the very idea that an earlier state can be reinstated as such is an illusion. Furthermore in the sense in which the infantile neurosis is still alive in the present it will be manifested in the present and does not require special measures to bring it to life. By the very fact that a regression beyond what the patient begins the treatment with has been induced, the regression cannot be a simple reinstatement of the past. What one should seek in analysis is not a level of regression beyond that which characterizes the patient's pathology, but a drawing into awareness of the regressive manifestations which up to that point have been expressed in disguise.
>
> [Gill, 1984a, p. 169]

The analyst can induce a regressive experience in the patient. But an induced state, simply by virtue of being 'induced,' is a different from the original non-induced state of mind. A pure reinstatement of an earlier state is therefore impossible. Nonetheless, Gill retains the concept of regression. The analyst should not induce regression, but work with the patient to uncover the disguised regressive manifestations still operative in the present.

There is implied, in Gill's perspective, a hierarchy of mentation from the regressive to the mature. He does not outline the hierarchy. He simply asserts that regressive mentation can outlive its original infantile state and persist in disguise in later mature states. There is an unarticulated value judgment here—a judgment about what characterizes infantile versus mature mentation—regardless of when said mentation occurs in the lifespan. The latent morality of maturity gets taken up later in the radical critique.

Stolorow, Brandchaft, and Atwood (1987) have outlined a regression perspective similar to Gill's later view. They use of the term 'archaic' organizing principles to indicate something like what Gill meant in 1984 by 'regressive' mentation irreducible to its origin point. They suggest that the adult's archaic mentation is related to the archaic mentation of childhood. But the former is not identical with the latter. If they *were* identical, then infant observation would, they hold, be able to demonstrate a stronger likeness.

They note, for example, that, in the adult patient, a dependent clinginess to maternal figures is often held to indicate a regression to an early phase of mother–infant symbiosis. But infancy research indicates, they counter-argue, that there is a normative alternation between moments of oneness with the mother and moments of disengagement (Stern, 1983; Beebe, 1986). These findings suggest that there is no continuous or prolonged period of normative mother–infant symbiosis. The adult patient's symbiotic wishes or fantasies "may be related to an early developmental period, but what the adult imagines, yearns for, or enacts is not identical to what is typical of the young child" (p. 31).

They allow for the continued use of the term 'regression' to indicate the emergence of archaic organizing principles in the present. The emergence of the archaic can serve defensive or restorative aims (see Chapter 1). But,

> in neither case can the patient be said to have actually retrogressed to an infantile period. We can only say that the patient's experiences . . . are being shaped by archaic organizing principles, either for the purpose of defense, or in order to resume a developmental process that had become stalled.
>
> (p. 32)

The Radical Critique

A more radical critique of the term *regression* has developed, with more recent origins, in the writings of Mitchell (1988), Inderbitzin and Levy (2000), and Wachtel (2003, 2008).

Like Stolorow, Brandchaft, and Atwood (see above), Mitchell (1988) argues for a distinction between the actual experience of infancy and the adult's experience of himself as a baby. The first is an immediate reality. The second is a symbolic experience, historically derivative of a real infancy, but firmly nested in the adult's present relational configurations. "The probably universal experience of oneself as a baby," he writes, "sometimes with playful delight, sometimes with shame and horror, does not reflect a direct reliving, a contact with one's deepest core, an expression of one's inner structural composition" (p. 150). Rather, it "reflects a pattern of symbolizing . . . adult experience in a form which draws its definitions and meanings from past and present relational configurations." One must wonder, then, what it means when the experience of oneself as a baby (or, alternatively, the experience of the other as a baby) emerges in the patient's or analyst's mind. We might regard it not as a regression, but as an event in the relational field.

Inderbitzin and Levy (2000) argue, in a more direct critique of regression, that the term is irredeemably flawed and should be discarded. They propose that 'regressive' shifts are better understood as non-regressive 'transformations' between modes of functioning. Each mode has an origin point and continues to develop across the phases of life. To reactivate a given mode is not to regress to the origin point. It is, rather, to reactivate a configuration of motives, defenses and adaptations nested fully in the here-and-now.

It follows, from their argument, that one could trace the development of so-called infantile or archaic modes through their development into their relatively mature present forms. To equate the former with the latter would amount to a genetic fallacy (Hartmann, 1955). It would ignore the mode's internal development. It would, moreover, neglect the mode's new function and significance in the contemporary internal and interpersonal worlds.

The 'deepest,' most 'primitive,' and most 'infantile' psychic structures develop and enter integratively into the emergent nexus of mental configurations in the present life phase. No one can make a pure return to an unmodified phase or mode of infantile organization.

A Magnet Beneath Iron Filings

We cannot, however, discard the term *regression*, in spite of its problems, without considering its clinical-theoretical utility. What function does it serve? Why has it lasted so long?

Mitchell (1988) argues, I think rightly, that it has served a hermeneutic function: It helps the psychoanalyst to organize the buzzing confusion of his immediate clinical encounter with the analysand into a circumscribed set of known categories, concepts and story lines:

> Whereas the analysand as adult appears to be operating in an obscure and puzzling fashion, viewing the analysand as child often helps us to organize the pieces and fragments of the analysand's experience into coherent, understandable patterns.
>
> (p. 127)

> The picture of the analysand-as-child orders the analytic data like the organizing impact of a magnet beneath a paper of scattered iron filings.
>
> (p. 128)

The hermeneutic pay-off of this imagery, in organizing the data, and ostensibly rendering the adult patient more understandable, explains, I suggest, the reluctance of many to give up the term *regression*. It has its flaws. But it seems to help.

It is important, to avoid confusion, to clarify the way in which I am using the term *hermeneutics*. I define it, in the tradition of Schleiermacher (1838), as "the art of understanding" (p. 5). The work of understanding proceeds, as Schleiermacher wrote of textual interpretation, through infinite iterations of a circular movement between part and whole. "Knowledge is always in this apparent circle," he wrote, "each particular can only be understood via the general, of which it is a part, and vice versa" (p. 24). To understand the analysand's thought, feeling or action is, therefore, to grasp its contextual function and significance in his internal world and, more broadly, in the present relational field.

We engage in the circular art of interpretation not as neutral observers, but as participant observers who exert conscious and unconscious influence. This does not have to be a crisis; it can be an opportunity. The analyst strives (imperfectly) to recognize the hindering effects of his 'fore-having,' 'fore-sight,' and 'fore-conception' (Heidegger, 1927, p. 153), or his 'prejudice' and 'fore-meanings' (Gadamer, 1960, p. 269), on his encounter with the alterity of the other. He avows, at the same time, and on a deeper level, that his biases and prejudices delimit the horizon of an historical perspective in which he is inextricably embedded. They are the positive condition of any understanding he achieves.

Some analysts, who use the term *hermeneutics* as a loose synonym for *social constructivism*, view the former as incompatible with the very act of metapsychological theorizing. The argument is that, if analytic insight never leads to anything deeper than a relative, co-constructed truth—a truth with subjective validity for the dyad, but no claim to objective truth—then it would be an epistemological mistake to cobble together such relativistic understandings into anything that would resemble a universal theory of mental functioning.

This is not, however, an inevitable conclusion. I adopt Habermas' (1968) alternative view of metapsychology as a 'metahermeneutics' (p. 254). It is an abstract system that represents, in short-hand, a tradition of understanding emergent from the clinical encounter. It amalgamates the experience of clinicians, working over many decades, into a system of beliefs, assumptions and practices that serve, in turn, to inform new iterations of hermeneutic immersion. As such, it constitutes a tradition—or perhaps more accurately an array of overlapping traditions—that shapes, but can fully predict or determine, the new understandings that we discover/create in daily work with new patients.

Ricoeur (2012) proposes a hermeneutics circle that runs back and forth in between the analyst's theories (and, I would add, the patient's theories) and the real-time processes of understanding and working through. A 'vicious circle' emerges, he asserts, when verification in one domain is mistaken as a condition for verification in another domain: if, for instance, the aesthetic satisfaction of theoretical coherence supplants the practical aim of working through issues and conflicts. I suggest that a generative circle emerges, by contrast, when the analyst's theory helps him implicitly or explicitly to understand his patients in a manner that helps them. The immediate hermeneutic and pragmatic utility of a theoretical idea or belief therefore serves as a check on the validity of the theory in question.

To return to the matter at hand, the metaphor of the baby, and the interdependent notion of regression, might have lasted so long in psychoanalytic thinking in part because of their hermeneutic utility. They help us to make sensible an array of adult experiences and behaviors that would otherwise appear nonsensical.

The history of psychoanalysis has shown, among other things, that it is impossible (and probably undesirable) to conceptualize the mind without recourse to metaphor. It is essential to remember, however, that our metaphorical babies *are* constructions. They cannot be observed, as such, in unmediated empirical reality. Different schools of thought have, after all, posited different, equally plausible 'babies' to organize infant observations and explain the problems of older patients. The Freudian baby, for example, is driven by powerful sexual and aggressive instincts that propel him through a series of unconscious 'danger situations' (Freud, 1926). The Kohutian baby, by contrast, is motivated by a primary striving for selfobject experiences of mirroring, idealization and twinship (Kohut, 1971, 1977). Self-object trauma results, for him, in drive-like sexual and aggressive strivings. The data for both babies is the same. But the causal theory is different. What is primary in one model is derivative and/or pathological in the other.

I do not mean to suggest that psychoanalytic theory lacks an evidence base in infant observation. I am arguing, however, that our theories organize such observational data—and amalgamate it with the 'regressive' experience of older patients—to create a picture of infancy that, in turn, will explain the adult's issues. The result is a hermeneutic circle in which the adult's problems are 'found' in the babies, and the problems of babies are then 'rediscovered' in the adult.

If we remain within the realm of metaphor, this can be a generative hermeneutic circle. (The adult's mind is like, *and unlike*, an infant's.) An evocative comparison, it can inspire new directions of inquiry, highlighting convergence and divergence, avoiding the literal equation of adult and infant selves.

But if the metaphorical comparison devolves into a literal equation, the hermeneutic circle becomes a vicious one. It then appears as if empirical evidence from the adult's unconscious proves it to be infantile. It looks as if there were a literal undeveloped child-self within the adult. But in actuality, we have simply pre-judged the unconscious as such. The 'evidence' simply reflects the manifestation of wishes, phantasies and defenses predefined as 'infantile' in our theory.

In taking the metaphor of the baby too literally, we forget what was implicit in its construction: that we constructed the 'baby' to house the adult's problems. We can deconstruct this baby, then, to show that his problems are not inherently infantile, but, rather, lifespan problems with iterations across the life cycle.

The Depths of the Unconscious

The vicious circle described above often involves another metaphor: psychic depth. The psychoanalytic metaphor of depth originated in Freud's depiction of the mind as an archeological dig site. In the *Studies on Hysteria* (Freud & Breuer, 1893–95), Freud likened the investigation of the mind to excavation of a 'buried city.' The investigator attempts to 'penetrate' the 'deeper layers' of memory (p. 139). The metaphor of depth survived the many developments in his thinking. In 1937, near the end of his life, he wrote:

> [The analyst's] work of construction, or, if it is preferred, of reconstruction, resembles to a great extent an archeologist's excavation of some dwelling-place that has been destroyed and buried or of some ancient edifice . . . just as the archeologist builds up the walls of the building from the foundations that have remained standing, determines the number and position of the columns from depressions in the floor and reconstructs the mural decorations and paintings from the remains found in the debris, so does the analyst proceed when de draws his inferences from the fragments of memories, form the associations and from the behavior of the subject of the analysis.
>
> [Freud, 1937b, p. 259]

One could interpret 'deep' to mean 'fundamental.' Deep mentation refers, then, to those desires, affects, phantasies and defenses most essential in structuring our experience of self and others. This interpretation makes no judgment about the onset time of deep mentation.

One could, however, going even further, interpret the archeological metaphor to mean that the earliest relics/memories lie deepest in the earth/psyche. We are then left with a problematic three-step equation: the deepest = the earliest = the most fundamental mentation.

Wachtel (2003) problematizes the space-time connection implicit in the metaphor of depth. "As one digs further down," he writes, "one finds the traces of earlier and earlier civilizations" (p. 8). The earlier = deeper equation is problematic, he argues, because it privileges infancy, while minimizing later development. Here the vicissitudes of latency, adolescent and adult development inevitably become 'superficial' and less important. It the history the field, a variety of theorists (e.g., Ferenczi, Klein, Winnicott,

Balint, Kohut and Hartmann) went back earlier and earlier into the childhood and even the womb. With a few notable exceptions (e.g., Erikson), major theorists paid less attention to adolescent and adult development. After all, who wants to stay on the 'surface'?

Like Mitchell, Wachtel argues that we have relegated to the theoretical baby themes that, in fact, remain important sources of conflict and struggle across the life cycle. Wachtel (2003, 2008) challenges us to consider the questions we don't ask because we implicitly perceive the patient's suffering through the lens of the depth metaphor. If we assume that childhood desires and phantasies are frozen, like wooly mammoths, in the depths of the psyche, we will be less likely to ask why they persist in the present. A countless number of childhood phantasies, he notes, drop out or change over time. If a pattern of mentation endures, we must, therefore, consider what here-and-now forces sustain, reinforce and perhaps alter its shape and function in present lived experience. It is insufficient to assume that it persists merely because it is buried deep in the earth of the mind and is thereby protected against the corroding effects of weather and climate.

The Morality of Maturity

As Ferenczi (1938) and Kohut (1984) taught us, we falsely attribute merger wishes to the child that are, in fact, normative and pervasive through all phases of the lifespan (see Chapter 5). The radical critique of regression extends this point beyond merger strivings to other lifespan phenomena—strivings and defenses—housed in a construction of childhood. Children *do* evidence these phenomena. But so do normal adults.

Mitchell (1988) argues that by locating vulnerable and unsettling desires in a metaphorical child (the child within the adult), we defend an image of maturity 'anemic' in its denial of passion, spontaneity and human fragility (p. 154). We uphold a self-protective (and self-deceptive) morality of maturity: Children are selfish, impulsive, needy, irrational and violent; adults are patient, rational, independent and socially constructive. If the adult exhibits the former qualities, it is really his inner child breaking out.

Psychoanalysis teaches us nothing, however, if not that all humans, young and old, healthy and sick, exhibit interwoven constructive and destructive phantasies and behaviors. We can all be rational and intensely irrational at the same time. We are all dependent. (Even those of us who function most 'independently.') We win an empty moral victory by projecting the unwanted aspects of adult experience into an infant-as-container. The adult's belief in his moral superiority is a narcissistic defense to be analyzed.

We find an instance of this morality, for instance, in Coen's (2000) defense of the term *regression*. Coen argues that the term regression, in spite of its flaws, is clinically useful and should therefore be retained. He warns analysts to be mindful of their own regressive wishes to relinquish their 'responsible,' 'differentiated' position and join with the patient in 'childlike relatedness.' The analyst is mature, responsible and independent (barring occasional and unfortunate, if inevitable, lapses); the patient is childish and merger-hungry.

Coen understands 'growth' as the achievement of 'maximum autonomy,' 'separateness' and 'competence' (p. 786). This traditional ego psychological position runs counter to a growing inter-school consensus that dependency is a lifelong feature of the human condition (Fairbairn, 1941; Kohut, 1984; Mitchell, 1988). Merger wishes, for instance, are just human (Kohut, 1984). They do not necessarily run counter to health or maturity. They can enter into the nexus of pathological or healthy psychological mental states. The impulse to locate them in the child is a prime example of the defense in question.

Interestingly, Coen's paper points the way out of this problem. He rejects the use of the term *regression* to designate any mode of relating, no matter how 'infantile,' if it promotes growth. "I regard as progressive," he writes, "despite their infantile nature, any childlike longings for an object relationship in which one can further develop oneself" (p. 793). In this sentence, he decouples the infantile and the regressive. The infantile can be progressive if it is growth oriented. A mental state is 'regressive' here only if it resists progress.

The real issue at stake is a question: How does the analytic couple understand, work toward and collude against growth? Growth might mean a greater freedom within the limits of one's dependencies. It might, alternatively, entail the deconstruction of a defensive illusion of autonomy and a greater acceptance of one's reliance on significant others. We can retain an interest in growth (the meaning of growth, our resistance to growth etc.) without framing the question in the form of an imperative to 'grow up.' It is possible to grow as an adult without pretending one is growing out of an internal childhood.

The Metaphor of the Machine

If revisit to Arlow and Brenner's (1964) clarification and defense of the term *regression*, we find one last essential metaphor: the metaphor of the mind as a machine. The mind is imagined as a machine with isolatable parts and functions. The machine-as-whole never regresses. Only certain parts or functions regress.

This logic might appear to rescue the concept of regression. We can, it suggests, isolate regressed functions without reducing them to their origins (genetic fallacy); we can inquire, instead, into their function in the here-and-now machine. We can explore how the present machine reinforces a reliance on regressed functions (avoiding the infantocentrism of the depth metaphor). We can reject the imagery of the patient as a child (morality of maturity), because, while certain functions regress, the machine-as-a-whole does not. The machine-as-a-whole—and therefore the patient—is always an adult machine.

The machine solution comes, however, at a high price. It reinforces, as Schafer (1976) argues, a picture of the psyche as a collection of anthropomorphized forces and functions. Behind the machine, there is always a person: the subject who operates the machine. The person, or subject, is an indivisible existential agent. Any attempt to divide him into functions presupposes a new agent behind those functions who operates them.

Consider, for example, a patient who represses hostile feelings toward her analyst and expresses them in the symbolic form of an arguing couple (Hinshelwood, 2008). The analyst suggests a transference link. The patient then appears to split off and annihilate the feelings. No longer represented in a symbolic form, the feelings are simply 'shredded' (p. 512).

One might be inclined to say, if we follow the machine-metaphor, that there was an ego regression from repression (which Klein [1930] considered a mature defense) to splitting (which Klein considered more infantile). Not all of the patient's ego functions regressed. Presumably many of her more mature defenses and adaptions remained operative.

But this reproduces a demonology of functions: Some ego functions behave regressively; others behave maturely. Behind the demonology, there is a person running the show. The person unconsciously represses her hostile feelings and, then, under increased pressure, splits them off and annihilates them. "At first, my patient had," Hinshelwood writes, "used a chance occurrence of the arguing couple to substitute for her bad feelings.

Later she annihilated the feelings." The agent is a holistic 'she,' not a part function.

From this viewpoint, the whole person (the 'she') splits off her hostility. If the whole person is not regressed (and the machine metaphorists would agree she isn't), then the splitting is not a regressive act. An adult agent, with a lifespan history, undertakes this action. If we had longitudinal data, we could, at best, compare her use of splitting as an infant to her use of splitting as an adult with an aim to determine the similarities and differences.

In this way the machine-metaphor re-inscribes the genetic fallacy. It isolates a function that appears similar to an infantile mechanism. It proceeds as if the function were operating in an infantile mode independent of the other mature functions of the machine. The metaphor thereby obscures the fact that there is a developed adult who operates even the ostensibly infantile function and thereby gives it a new psychic significance.

It is worth nothing, before leaving this example that, Hinshelwood arrives, by a different path, at a similar conclusion: that splitting is no more infantile that repression. 'Is splitting,' he asks, "a defense of an ego that is less mature than one using repression?" (p. 515.) "The clinical material did *not* confirm this prediction. Both defense mechanisms can be used by the *same* ego (in the same analytic relationship) on the same day."

In rejecting the term *regression*, we therefore reject the genetic fallacy, the infantocentrism of the depth metaphor and the morality of maturity. In further rejecting the machine-metaphor solution, we reject the anthropomorphization of isolated mental functions and the subtle way in which it re-inscribes the very genetic fallacy it attempts to avoid.

Chapter 3

The Person as Agent

The theory of regression, and its conservative critics, rely on a model of the mind in which one can distinguish infantile residues or functions from the mature aspects of the personality. This vision of the mind breaks down upon recognition that early- and later-acquired functions are inextricably melded in the person's adaptation to the present phase of life.

The proper subject of psychoanalytic inquiry is, I argue, not the isolated wish, need, defense, or phantasy, but the person: the irreducible agent of his experience in the present (Schafer, 1976). He thinks, feels and acts out of the whole of his development. We can always zero in, as a thought exercise, on the processes in his inner world which remind us, in isolation, of those at play in child development. But it is just a thought exercise. In lived reality these very processes have entered into a new, emergent way of being.

The idea of an 'irreducible' agent might raise concern for those who think it is necessary to divide the mind into separate agencies (e.g., id, ego and superego) to account for the phenomena of self-alienation, for example, the sense of being lived by unknown forces (Freud, 1923). But the unity of the person does not negate the sense of being in conflict with oneself. Nor does it negate the sense of being driven to act in ways one does not understand. The person, in this particular sense of the term, is the human agent who has always been implicit in the anthropomorphized agencies of classical psychoanalytic metapsychology.

Perhaps the central activity of the person is to organize and make sense of his experience. I argue, following Klein (1976) and Gill (1983), that psychoanalysis studies not drives per se, but the way the person represents his motives and the meaning he gives them. The important point is that the act of representation itself is always a here-and-now event.

The implicit critique of drive theory might suggest an interpersonal-relational model. Mitchell (1988), for instance, read Klein (1976) as trending in a relational direction. I reject, however, what I consider the false (but popular) dichotomy between drive and relational psychology. Human motives, which, like all mentation, are grounded in neurological action potentials, enter into psychoanalytic discourse only when one-person, that is, the analysand, represents them to another, that is, the analyst, in a relational context.

The Implicit Subject

The mechanistic model of the mind, to which Arlow and Brenner (1964) appealed, serves a problematic rhetorical purpose. It allows us to admit that the machine-as-a-whole is always a present phenomenon, while preserving the logic of regression in the imagery of the isolated infantile part or function (as if the part could be assessed in isolation). To reject the logic of regression, one must rule out this particular effort to save it.

Arlow and Brenner draw, in their solution, on the structural model of the mind (Freud, 1923). Freud had recognized, by the 1920s, that the subject does not consciously repress his wishes. The analysand is unaware not only of his impulses but of his defenses against them. And not only is he unaware of his defenses, but he resists being made aware of them. The recognition forced Freud to revise his earlier model of the mind. In his prior model, the preconscious system repressed unconscious impulses (Freud, 1915). But the preconscious is, by definition, that to which the conscious mind can attend *if* it pays attention. To explain the resistance to defense analysis, Freud replaced the preconscious system with the ego: an executive agency with an unconscious sector that operates the defenses. The ego could thus observe itself and yet resist awareness of its unconscious functions.

The ego psychological tradition subsequently elaborated the ego into a complex machine (see, for instance, Hartmann, Kris, & Loewenstein, 1946). The ego machine, in this model, yokes together functions and subfunctions with distinct developmental lines (Freud, 1965). The functions operate in sync to harness, manage and discharge the energies of the id. It is this imagery to which Arlow and Brenner appeal in their assertion that, in any given regression, only certain mental functions—not the entire system—have regressed.

Over the second half of the twentieth century, a diverse collection of critics emerged to argue, for various reasons, that psychoanalysis studies not *functions* but *persons* in action. One of the most powerful group of critics appeared in 1970s American ego psychology. The proponents—Roy Schafer, Merton Gill, George Klein and Donald Spence—argued, in an explicit rejection of their own ego psychological training, that psychoanalysis cannot, and should not, reduce the subject to an energy-discharging machine.

Schafer (1976) argues, in perhaps the most thorough such critique, that we have misunderstood our own subject matter. Psychoanalysts, he writes, "deal essentially with [their analysand's] reasons, emphases, choices, and the like," and yet, "they have traditionally made it their objective to translate these subjective contents and these actions into the language of functions, energies, and so forth" (p. 103). The translation act, by which we aspire to a dispassionate scientific language, distorts and confuses our inquiry. We never observe an isolated energy or function. Rather, we observe persons who defensively distort the very wishes and strivings that animate their every waking action.

About 25 years prior Fairbairn (1952) had advanced a similar critique of drive theory. The libidinal wish, he argued, always implies a wishing ego. Our erotic impulses are simply the "forms of activity in which the life of ego structures consists" (p. 87). Psychoanalysis tends to speak of 'the libido' as if one could isolate the wish from the wisher. But that is a scientific fallacy—one that his object-relations theory aimed to correct. The problem, in light of Schafer's critique, is that Fairbairn proceeded to posit five dynamic structures.[1] Schafer leads us to recognize that, behind any such constellation, there is, in fact, one agent: the person who brings it all together in each action.

Schafer did not critique the concept of regression. But he helps lay the foundation for a critique. He shows that, behind any isolated function, there is always an irreducible person. Unlike the machine, he person cannot be parsed into mature and regressive functions (see Chapter 2). He—the whole agent—is implied in even the most childish actions. He—in all of his developmental sophistication—is always behind the figurative gears.

Schafer proposes a simple, but powerful strategy for revision: We can reframe ego psychological tenets in terms of an irreducible person, or subject, who acts on himself and his world. We must first locate the person behind our discourse on anthropomorphic energies and psychic structures. Consider Freud's (1917c) portrayal of the ego in melancholia:

> The analysis of melancholia now shows that the ego can kill itself only if, owing to the return of the object-cathexis, it can treat itself as an object—if it is able to direct against itself the hostility which relates to an object. (p. 251)

Or consider Freud's (1926) depiction of conflict upon regression to sadistic forms of libidinal expression:

> The ego will recoil with astonishment from promptings to cruelty and violence which enter consciousness from the id, and it has no notion that in them it is combating erotic wishes, including some to which it would not otherwise have taken exception. The overstrict superego insists all the more strongly on the suppression of sexuality, since this has assumed such repellent forms.
>
> (Freud, 1926, p. 115)

The id, ego and superego are portrayed as agents with their own affects, intentions, interpretations and choices. There is, in the act of anthropomorphization, Schafer argues, an implicit recognition of the limitations of mechanistic language to capture the subject as agent:

> We are all aware that Freud did not adhere consistently to the scientific model on which he had pinned his theoretical hopes. While using it, he 'anthropomorphized' it. In doing so he made some of his most memorable statements—for example, when he spoke of the superego as the heir of the Oedipus complex, and of the ego's serving three masters, or letting itself die, or deforming itself. Freud often spoke in this way of the psychic structures, the topographic systems, the primary and secondary processes, the great principles, and the instinctual drives and energies: he spoke of all of these as if they were purposive, meaning-creating, choice-making, action oriented entities, which is to say, as if they were minds within the mind, or homunculi.
>
> (Schafer, 1976, p. 104)

Schafer welcomes the anthropomorphizing trend in Freud's theorizing as an implicit sign that Freud could not adequately express his insights through the language of drives and functions. Behind the psychic structures, there appears a subject: a conscious and unconscious agent of experience. "There was a person," Schafer writes, "loose in the apparatus, a mastermind working the mechanism . . . the mover of the mental apparatus" (p. 110).

By replacing mechanisms/functions with persons in action, psychoanalysis can, Schafer argues, pull its insights from their false packaging in mechanistic jargon and recognize them in their proper light—the light of a humanistic discourse on agency and choice. He terms his discourse 'action language.' It is a descriptive language of persons in action.[2]

Freud's asserted, as mentioned above, that, in a libidinal regression to sadistic modes of expression,

> The ego will recoil with astonishment from promptings to cruelty and violence which enter consciousness from the id, and it has no notion that in them it is combating erotic wishes, including some to which it would not otherwise have taken exception. The overstrict superego insists all the more strongly on the suppression of sexuality, since this has assumed such repellent forms.
>
> (Freud, 1926, p. 115)

We can restate the assertion to read:

> The patient recoils with astonishment from his cruel and violent impulses, without realizing their erotic nature. He becomes overstrict in insisting, all the more strongly, albeit unconsciously, on repressing his impulses, since they now emerge in such repellent forms.

The reframe highlights the person in action. It can, of course, be taken too far. It is unnecessary to purge our discourse of metaphorical agentic structures. It is important simply to recognize that, in our metaphorical use of agentic structures, we are describing an irreducible agentic person. The person acts as a whole. If we forget the metaphor and buy into the literal picture of the mind-as-machine, we fall into a host of errors previously mentioned.

Schafer's critique is not limited to Freudian metapsychology. It opens a common language—that of persons in action—through which to compare and contrast alternative models. Schafer (1976) suggests, for instance, that self-psychology too searches, in the construct of the 'self,' for a humanistic psychology of persons (not machines). The problem, for Schafer, is that the *self* becomes another organization of anthropomorphic functions. Self-psychologists Stolorow and Atwood (1984) arrive at a similar place. "We have found it important," they write, "to distinguish sharply between the concept of the self as a psychological structure and the concept of the person as an experiencing subject and agent who initiates action" (p. 29). The person is the agent; the self an organization of experience. One might, by implication, compare the Freudian *person* to the Kohutian *person*. The gain, which we cannot explore here, is a common ground for dialogue and debate.

One might extend the argument further to cover recent neurological theories of motivation. Psychoanalysts Solms and Turnbull (2002) have drawn, for instance, on Panksepp's (1998) research in affective neuroscience to posit a contemporary drive theory. They go beyond the dual drive model to suggest four "basic-emotion command systems." The *seeking system*, located in the ventral tegmental area, uses dopamine to arouse and sustain interest in the world. It includes the *lust* subsystem, which generates feelings of 'pleasurable delight,' when the seeking system has attained the object of interest. The *rage system* is triggered by the medial nucleus of the amygdaloid complex and runs through the bed nucleus of the stria terminalis and anterior, ventromedial and perifornical hypothalamus. It is activated by frustration when goal-directed actions are thwarted. The *fear system*, centered in the lateral and central nuclei of the amygdaloid complex, generates feelings of fear and initiates the flight response. The *panic system*, which relies on endogenous opiods, is centered in the anterior cingulate gyrus and runs into the bed nucleus of the stria terminalis, the preoptic hypothalamus and the ventral tegmental area. It is distinct from the fear system in generating the panic of separation and loss.

It would lead beyond the present critique to evaluate the four systems in their own right. I use them merely to illustrate the continued relevance of Schafer's critique. To apply Schafer's action language here is to point out the simple, but important, point that the clinical psychoanalyst does not study any of these neurological systems directly. He does not, for instance, study the seeking system per se. He studies the *person* who seeks. The person—the irreducible subject who emerges out of a lifespan history—is always the focus of inquiry. Suppose the adult analysand revived a seeking-pattern neurologically identical to a childhood pattern. The analytic process would not map the neurological system directly. Rather, it would explore meaning the person makes in the present of whatever he now seeks. It would not be a regression because, although the present neurological system would be identical with its childhood precursor, the meaning of the object sought—in the context of the person's holistic life context—would be something new.

The pay-off, for our purposes, is that action language, as mentioned in Chapter 2, highlights the falsity of a mechanistic division of the mind into regressed and mature functions. The machine-metaphor admits that the mind/machine as a whole operates in the present. It preserves the theory of regression by positing that only certain functions regress. Action language disallows that parsing move. The irreducible person performs every function. He brings his full history and present potential to bear on whatever he does.

We can, at best, study the similarity between his past and present actions. But we must inquire equally into the disjunction and, amidst repetition, into the potential for novelty.

Present Meaning

The psychoanalyst engages, through associations and fragmented narratives, with the person who has already represented, organized and made sense of the experience he brings. To study the person in action is, in essence, to study the meaning he makes of his daily life. The point, for my argument, is that meaning-making is always a here-and-now activity.

The work of George Klein (1976) provides an entry point into this portion of the discussion. He draws an instructive distinction between the drive-discharge model in Freudian theory and the implicit 'clinical theory,' which is more nuanced, in his clinical writing. The drive-discharge theory, to begin, presents the libido as a quantifiable bodily force. The force finds mental representation in an instinct (Freud, 1905). The instinct seeks discharge by cathecting ideas, memories, dream images, symptoms, ego and superego structures and external objects. At the heart of this model, we find a core assumption that, "the source of all activity in the organism . . . is its tendency to deal with energic influxes of stimuli and to discharge them, to reduce the tensions" (Klein, 1976, p. 73).

The problem with the drive-discharge model, from the perspective of a regression critique, is that the libido has, by age five or six, passed through all of the major posited erotogenic zones. The original fixations, of which all later mental life is thought to be derivative, have been formed. A hermeneutic circle emerges in which infancy is always bedrock. An oral wish becomes, for instance, 'evidence' of a regression to the oral phase. The drive itself lacks the qualitative texture we need to show what is new about the wish.

The clinical theory, by contrast, inquiries into the varied subjective meanings of lust and love. The analyst and analysand explore the qualitative "properties peculiar to sexuality, upon the values and meanings associated with sensual experiences in the motivational history of a person from birth to adulthood, upon how nonsexual motives and activities are altered when they acquire a sensual aspect, and vice versa" (Klein, 1976, p. 73). It seeks a qualitative texture that cannot but reflect the here-and-now context.

The clinical theory does not deny the quantitative factor in sexual attraction. However, it takes as its subject not the quantitative force per se, but its qualitative texture in a lifespan context. The interest in meaning is implicit in Freud's (1905) contention that the instinct is the mental representation of a bodily force—a phantasy—and not its direct manifestation. Implicit in our unconscious sexual phantasies are feelings of comfort, power, worth, access, exclusion and so on. These cognitive-affective meanings—and their associative link with other meanings—evolve, as few would deny, across the life cycle.

Not only does the person-as-a-whole initiate action; he also makes sense of his experience, consciously and unconsciously, in ways that reflect his embeddedness in the here and now. As long as we consider the emergence of an isolated wish or phantasy as evidence that the person has regressed to the phase or mental organization of its first manifestation, we will find ourselves trapped in a tautology in which we perpetually reconfirm the regressive nature of adult experience. This circle exemplifies the genetic fallacy. If we instead regard the wish or phantasy as a subjective phenomenon with a contemporary significance, we will find out not only what is historically bound, but also what might be different or novel about the person's experience of his wish in the present moment.

The critique of Freud's drive-discharge theory of sexuality can be extended to the narcissistic, borderline or schizoid patient's allegedly 'archaic' or 'primitive' attunement needs. If our theories pre-define as 'infantile' the lifelong human need for holding (Winnicott, 1945a,1945b), primary love or harmonious merger (Balint, 1968), mirroring and idealizing (Kohut, 1971, 1977) and so on, then we will find ourselves in another tautology. We will confirm again and again the adult patient's regressive longings whenever he expresses, in words or nonverbal actions, the lifespan needs we pre-judged to be infantile. We can escape from this tautology, if, as with sexual instincts, we explore the personal meaning of the needs in the present. We might wonder, for instance, what it means to be held or mirrored now. It then becomes clear that our basic needs—their significance, what they look like, what it means to meet or not meet them—evolve over a lifetime.

The Interpersonal-Relational Tradition

The relatively recent interest in the 'person,' grounded in a critique of mental mechanization, picks up on what has long been a central thread of interpersonal psychoanalysis. Sullivan (1953), for instance, in his chapter titled "The Infant as a Person," portrays the oral zone as a site not just of libidinal pleasure, but of interpersonal interaction and emergent personhood. When the nursing infant experiences the mother feeling pleased and being tender, he personifies his self-state in a nascent sense of 'Good-me.' When his actions create tension and evoke a 'forbidding' response, then he personifies his self-state in a nascent sense of 'Bad-me.' When his actions evoke in the parent (and consequently in himself) unthinkably disturbing affects—for example, silent dread, horror or loathing—he dissociates from what becomes 'Not-me': an unformulated smog of "poorly grasped aspects of living which will presently be regarded as dreadful" (p. 163).

It is not necessary, for the critique of regression, to adopt Sullivan's portrait of the psyche in all of its details. One need not, for instance, abandon a Freudian repression model of the mind for a contemporary Sullivanian dissociation model (Stern, 2003a, 2003b, 2011, 2015). I have argued elsewhere that the person can use both defenses (Rizzolo, 2016). By dissociation, he can keep apart subjectively incompatible feeling states. Meanwhile, within each feeling state, he can use repression to bury dangerous thoughts, feelings and wishes.

We find another early interpersonal resource in Erich Fromm's writing. Fromm (1991) argued, from a humanistic perspective, that the analyst should regard the patient as a 'person,' born with certain gifts, fighting against his handicaps, to make something of his life (p. 600). He urged analysts to look beyond Freud's (1937a) emphasis on quantitative instinctual factors (e.g., a strong/weak libido or death instinct) to the human person's innate capacity for vitality, courage and love of life. Fromm can only take us so far, however. At times his writing, in fact, epitomizes the patient-infantilization in question: "the patient must travel on two tracks . . . he must show himself as, experience himself as, the child, let us say, of two or three he is unconsciously, but he must at the same time also be an adult, responsible person who faces this part of himself" (Fromm, 1991, p. 591).

It is important, while recognizing these historical resources, to differentiate my argument from what I consider the mistaken dichotomy between drive and relational perspectives. The dichotomy derives from Greenberg and Mitchell (1983) and Mitchell's (1988) influential contributions, which, apart from this detail, have strongly influenced my argument. They assert a division between *drive models*, which study energy discharge, and *relational models*, which take the self–other unit as the object of psychoanalytic inquiry. Having constructed the division, they apply it to critique prior critics of Freud who did not, by their assessment, adequately reject drive psychology for relational psychology.

Mitchell's (1988) critique of George Klein illustrates the problem I find in this approach. He argues that Klein 'drifted' toward a relational theory of motivation, but perhaps out of loyalty to tradition, refused to replace the libido theory with a more fully relational model (p. 89). He moved toward such a model, Mitchell argues, in that he (a) rejected drive theory and (b) recognized the social meaning at play in shaping our sexual desires. But he mistakenly believed, according to Mitchell, that Freudian theory could endure such a move. To remove drive theory is, for Mitchell, to create an unacceptable explanatory vacuum. It becomes unclear what motivates the subject to engage with others.

A relational theory of motivation has the potential, in Mitchell's reading, to fill the vacuum. Mitchell (1988) proposes that the primary human motive is "to establish strong connections to others, in reality or in fantasy" (p. 91). Sexual desire is not a "pre-constituted push from within," but "a response or action within an interactive context" (p. 89). Sexual experience remains relevant because it proves an 'apt arena' for seeking and playing out various relational patterns: "discovery, penetration, dominance, surrender, control, longing, evasion, revelation, envelopment, merger, differentiation, and so on" (p. 91). He thus replaces the libido with a universal, non-drive motive to establish object relations.

Mitchell is right about the explanatory vacuum. The question is, Do we need to reject the very possibility of a 'drive' theory, or more simply, the asocial aspect of *Freud's* drive theory. I suggest that, if we reject the asocial nature of the Freudian drives, and replace it with a thoroughly social model of neurological motivation, then there is no reason to discard the basic possibility of a drive theory. As mentioned, Solms and Turnbull (2002) attempt this project. Their motivational systems are each thoroughly social. The seeking system, for instance, "does not appear to know what it is seeking" (p. 118). From birth onwards, the person relies on social interaction, which he internalizes and represents in memory, to shape and elicit what he seeks. Why must we choose, then, between a world of powerful endogenous forces and one of thorough-going relational immersion?

Mitchell (1988) wanted to reject the asocial aspect of Freudian drive theory in particular. But he perhaps draws too broad a contrast between drive and relational models in general. It is as if one could not have a relational drive theory. This either/or lacks the nuance of other passages in Mitchell's (1988) treatise. He writes elsewhere that "powerful biological surges in the phenomenology of sexual excitement" lead to a "sense of being 'driven'" (p. 103). He thus suggests a phenomenology of physiological forces. He returns, in this way, to the representation of the body in Freud's (1905) term 'instinct.' The essential point, for my argument, is that the person imbues his sexual desire—and a range of other embodied social motives—with ever-evolving relational meaning.

Thinking

What seems lacking in the discussion of personal meaning is a theory of meaning itself. It is unclear what we mean by *meaning* and how it fits into a depth model of the mind.

In the *Interpretation of Dreams* (1900) and later in "*Formulations on the Two Principles of Mental Functioning*" (1911), Freud developed a preliminary model of thinking. He suggested that internal needs disrupt the mind and prompt hallucinatory wish fulfillment. The hallucination fails to satisfy for long and leans into secondary process planning. The mind learns thereby to represent the world and to make adaptive changes.

This process marks the institution, alongside the pleasure principle, of the reality principle. The two principles operate, in harmony or disharmony, through the 'pleasure-ego' and the 'reality-ego.' The reality ego safeguards the pleasure principle in striving purposively for assured pleasure at a later time in accordance with real opportunities for satisfaction.

The process of thinking develops, in Freud's model, in the space of delay between wish and satisfaction. Thinking is, he asserts, "an experimental kind of acting" (Freud, 1911, p. 220). It conserves energy while the person plans, evaluates and seeks delayed gratification. It proceeds unconsciously by creating networks of imagistic ideational residues. These networks enter consciousness, but only in part, through connection with words.

Bion (1962), who elaborated Freud's model, distinguishes between 'beta-elements' (raw sensory experience that cannot be thought) and alpha-elements (beta-elements transformed by 'alpha-function' into the material of dreams and waking thought). He holds that alpha-function depends on a capacity for tolerating frustration. "A capacity for tolerating frustration," he writes, "enables the psyche to develop thought as a means by which the frustration that is tolerated is itself made more tolerable" (p. 112).

The development of frustration tolerance depends, in turn, on the infant's experience of the mother's 'reverie.' The infant projects beta-elements into the mother, who, in optimal development, contains and transforms them in her reverie into something more tolerable. "Normal development follows if the relationship between infant and breast permits the infant to project a feeling, say, that it is dying into the mother and to reintroject it after its sojourn in the breast has made it more tolerable to the infant psyche" (p. 116).

If there is a break down in mother's capacity for reverie, then the beta-elements will be left unmodified and are re-introjected in an unmanageable form by the infant psyche. "If the projection is not accepted by the mother," Bion writes, in continuation of his example, "the infant feels that its feeling that it is dying is stripped of such meaning as it has. It therefore reintrojects, not a fear of dying made more tolerable, but a nameless dread" (p. 116). The nameless dread must then be dealt with through new rounds of projection.

Ferro (1999a) elaborates Bion's system into a model of the dynamic unconscious. 'Sensory perceptions' (beta-elements) stream into the mind and are transformed into 'movie frames' (alpha-elements). "As these elements gradually come into being, they may," he writes, "be turned either up, in which case they form the system of consciousness, or down, forming the unconscious system" (pp. 45–46). The unconscious is made up of "face-down alpha-elements" and "undigested facts," another Bionian term, by which Ferro means, "accumulations of emotional or sensory-perceptual proto-tensions." The latter can be seen as "partly digested and metabolized beta-elements," or "balpha-elements."

"The human individual," Bion (1962) wrote, "is a political animal and cannot satisfy any emotional drive without expression of its social component" (p. 118). Ferro (1999b) bridges Bion's interest in group life with the Baranger's (1964) interest in the 'bi-personal field.' He distinguishes between the Freudian focus on factual historical relationships, the Kleinian focus on intrapsychic relationships, and the Bionian focus on the 'field,' that is, the "current emotional interrelationship between analyst and patient" (p. 2). Without denying the importance of factual history or of intrapsychic relationships, Ferro considers the patient's communication a signal of the functioning of the relational field.

The analytic field, like the infant–mother dyad, contains and transforms sensory and proto-emotion experience into the material of conscious and unconscious thought and phantasy. Breakdowns, signaled by the patient's evacuative communications, reflect field pathology.

Sullivan (1940) similarly argued, albeit from a different perspective, and without reference Freud's 'Two Principles,' that much of what psychoanalysis considers repressed is, in fact, unformulated. Unformulated experience is not thought about, not even not even unconsciously (Stern, 1983). It exists only in a state of potential: a vague and disturbing tendency of feeling, which gets stopped short, prior to verbal or imagistic formulation. The defense here is not repression, which operates on the formulated, but dissociation.

We find a point of contact between Bionian field theory and relational field theory in the overlapping concepts of beta-elements and unformulated experience. Stern (2015) writes:

> In both IRP [interpersonal-relational psychoanalysis] dissociation theory and In the BFT [Bionian field theory] theory of the transformation of mental contents . . . symbolic experience has yet to be constructed. . . . Symbolic experience is not yet shaped, or formed; it exists in either a primitive, unmentalized state . . . or as potential that has not yet been actualized in symbolic form. I have already mentioned that Ferro describes the creation of symbolic experience as 'alphabetization' or transformation. . . . I refer to it as the process of formulating experience.
>
> (p. 86)

The convergence of the two models suggests—without minimizing the generative differences—a mutually enriching dialogue on how meaning is constructed in the present field.

Stern (2015) suggests the relational and Bionian field models might differ not in their essential tenets, or principles, but in their historical origins and distinct cultural applications. The interpersonal-relational tradition, which originated in America, outside mainstream Freudian psychoanalysis, has focused on the deconstruction of the analyst's authority. The ubiquity of the field implies that he, too, is subject to forces beyond his control. A proper analysis extends to include the patient's experience of his unconscious participation (Hoffman, 1983; Aron, 1991). The Bionian tradition, by contrast, which grew up in Europe and South America, has been less interested in a critique of analytic authority. The analyst is trusted to receive and interpret patient projections in relative neutrality. It is plausible, although it cannot be pursued here, that American trends have fostered an analytic culture uniquely suspicious, on the world stage, of its own exercise of power.

Katz (2017), by contrast, considers the same difference a sign of theoretical-epistemological disagreement. In the Bionion model, the patient uses the analyst's alpha-function in order to think. The analyst, it implies, has "direct access . . . to the analysand's beta elements" (p. 136). He can thus metabolize the analysand's as-yet unmediated emotional experience. A great degree of authority is therefore invested in the analyst's alpha-function. In the relational model the analyst, by contrast, has no such direct access. He always understands from the vantage point of his subjective world or horizon (Stern, 2003a). Whatever he perceives he has already organized through implicit unconscious expectations. No one, by this model, could ever access an unmediated proto-emotional truth.

It might be possible to develop a critique of regression from either theoretical-epistemological position. The present critique, however, leans in favor of the relational perspective. The person, as I shall later argue, always acts of out a lifespan history to make sense of his present experience (see Chapter 5). By implication he brings the influence of past development to bear—in unconscious ways—on whatever he now confronts. In this regard the analyst is no different from the analysand. He cannot help but listen to the analysand from the unique vantage point of his own developmental history. Whatever he hears he has already organized according to his own acquired prejudices.

The proper focus of psychoanalytic inquiry is, then, the irreducible agent—the person—assumed in any psychoanalytic proposition. The person (not the isolated drive or need) lusts or strives for objects the significance of which reflects a meaning-making process. The constant process of shaping and reshaping meanings occurs in the relational field. The field supports/hinders they very act of thinking by which experience becomes meaningful. It is, therefore, to psychoanalytic models of the field that we turn in the next chapter.

Notes

1 These are the central ego, the internal saboteur, the libidinal ego, the rejecting object and the exciting object (Fairbairn, 1952, p. 105)

2 Schafer himself pursues it to a behaviorist extreme, considering affects as actions. We do not need to go that far. The main point here is that we study the person who emotes. We do not, for instance, study childlike emotions in isolation. The adult person who emotes in childlike ways still experiences as an adult. He has not regressed, and no isolated part of him has regressed, to a literal state of childhood affectivity. We implicitly recognize this fact in that we would not include him in a study of affect in actual children.

Chapter 4

The Field of Deferred Action

The psychoanalytic study of the person inevitably involves an inquiry into the present relational context in which he makes conscious and unconscious meaning of his experience. Without context, life would, as interpersonal and Bionian field theories attest, be meaningless.

A number of regression theorists do, in fact, pay attention to the interpersonal environment. Freud (1912–13, 1921), Bion (1961) and the Barangers and Baranger (1964) have written on irrational group and couple phantasy life. A separate but related trend explores the pre-Oedipal child's dependency on the parents, especially the mother, for holding, mirroring, soothing etc. (Hartmann, 1939; Winnicott, 1954a, 1954b; Balint, 1968; Kohut, 1971).

The theorists of regressive group function and those of the regressive pre-Oedipal dyad run into a tautology, however, outlined in Chapter 2, in which universal group processes and lifelong dependency needs, observable at all ages, are pre-determined to be infantile. Their re-occurrence in adulthood then counts as 'evidence' for a universal regressive trend. The tautology limits our ability to perceive novelty in the context of the familiar.

The interpersonal-relational and intersubjective traditions, with respective roots in Sullivan and Kohut, have done the most to conceptualize our immersion in interactional fields without falling back on regression theory to explain their often irrational or volatile nature. I argue for an integrative relational-intersubjective position in which the present field shapes the conscious and unconscious experience/psychic structure of the participants. The integration relies, within relational thought, on a synthesis of repression and dissociation models and, within intersubjectivity theory, on a revised view of projective identification, which, historically, the major proponents of the theory have rejected.

The relational field, to continue, becomes the site of an ongoing process of *Nachträglichkeit*, or deferred action: The residues of past experience are modified, reorganized, fleshed out, and endowed with new meaning/purpose in the immediate interaction. I draw on Klein's (1937) description of a stable and contented marriage to illustrate the normative process by which the current matrix re-contextualizes childhood attachments.

The emergence of child and adolescent characters, or representations, in an adult analysis constitutes a dramatic instance of deferred action in the analytic field. Instead of presuming an equation between the characters of the session and the patient's actual past self, we can consider them, in light of their historical precursors, to be novel products of the field. Their literal correspondence with the past is less relevant than their function in the present. I illustrate this phenomenon through Davies and Frawley's (1991) vivid portrayal of the 'child persona' in the psyche of the adult survivor of childhood sexual abuse.

The Regressive Field

Freud recognized that the mind—in all its unconscious depth—is embedded in social relationships. He speculated, in *Totem and Taboo* (1912–1913) and *Civilization and its Discontents* (1930), that a primal horde of brothers killed and devoured their jealous and violent father. They were left, he suggested, with a collective sense of guilt, which, over thousands of years, developed into the 'cultural superego' of our present society (1930, p. 141). Setting aside its speculative nature, one finds in this narrative a basic recognition of the intergenerational influence of group life on individual moral structure.

In *Group Psychology and the Analysis of the Ego* (1921), Freud defined a group as "a number of individuals who have put one and the same object [the leader] in the place of their ego-ideal and have consequently identified themselves with one another in their ego" (p. 116). If we consider Freud's (1923) later assertion that the ego develops through identification with lost objects, and the fact that all object-ties (and thus all lost objects) are embedded in groups, it becomes clear that, in Freud's theory, group relations must play an essential, if under-emphasized, role in the development and structuring of the psyche.

Bion (1961) expanded projective identification (Klein, 1946) from a one-person phantasy into an actual exchange between a projector and a receptor/container. This expansion underlies his theory of irrational group life. Every group, he argued, has both a rational-conscious task and an unconscious phantasy life that disrupts it. The primary mechanism of disruption is projective identification. Primitive anxieties lead to splitting and the projection of part objects into the receptor. The receptor is an individual who possesses the right 'valence,' a capacity to cooperate with the collective projection. The group then proceeds as if it has convened for the purpose of managing its anxiety via the receptor.

The group members behave as if they shared a basic assumption. They might, for instance, assume that they have met "in order to be sustained by a leader on whom [they] depend for nourishment, material and spiritual, and protection" (p. 147). They might assume that they have met "to fight something or to run away from it" (p. 152). Or they might indulge in 'pairing' phantasies, for example, in the idea that "either marriage or polyamory would end neurotic suffering, that group therapy would revolutionize society, that the coming season will be more agreeable, or that some new kind of community should be developed" (p. 151). Pairing include the idea of a messiah: "a person or idea that will save the group—in fact from feelings of hatred, destructiveness, and despair." The preservation of hope depends, however, on the fact that the Messiah never comes, never disappoints.

The Barangers and Baranger (1964) argue that a 'bipersonal,' or 'intersubjective' field is constituted by reciprocal projective identifications and emergent unconscious 'couple' fantasies. The fight/flight fantasy in Bion's groups illustrates their meaning of a shared field fantasy. It exists within the field. One could not locate it 'in' an individual outside of the field. In the analytic situation, like in the group setting, the analyst and analysand respond unconsciously to each other and contribute to the emergence of a shared fantasy life.

The patient is determined, the Barangers and Baranger (1964) write, to keep certain material outside of the analytic situation: special object relationships, perverse activities, an ideology etc. Such resistances manifest in breaches of the fundamental rule to free associate. If the analyst becomes complicit, there develops a 'bastion' in the field. In these cases, "a sector of the field crystallizes, comprising the patient's resistance and the analyst's counter-resistance, unconsciously communicated and operating together, while on another separate level an apparently normal communication goes on" (p. 9). This is 'field pathology.' By interpreting at the 'point of urgency' (where the couple fantasy breaches the manifest content), the analyst and patient can re-integrate the disowned mentation and, in dissolving the bastion, re-open the field for new transformations in experience.

Ferro (1999a) finds a point of convergence in Bion and the Barangers work in the shared idea that, in the analytic field, the analyst's mental functioning in part structures, and is in part structured by, the patient's mental functioning. While the Barangers recommend 'strong' interpretations—marked by explicit imputation of unconscious phantasy content—Ferro and Bion, however, favor 'open-ended' or 'unsaturated' interpretations—less certain inferences, aimed not at decoding, but at the creation of new meaning. The strong interpretation presupposes a formed unconscious phantasy, waiting to be decoded. The open-ended interpretation, by contrast, presupposes a more fluid unconscious phantasy life: one that consists of partly formed phantasy, with many un-thought or undreamed elements, the co-articulation of which constitutes the analytic work.

The difference here does not imply an incompatibility. One might see the Barangers as focused strictly on what Bion and Ferro would regard as alpha element phantasies. Their strict focus does not, in principle, discourage an expanded focus, which Bion introduced, and which Ferro has championed, to theorize the un-thought realm of beta-elements. The unconscious consists ultimately of both formulated and unformulated elements.

Freud, Bion and the Barangers, among others, help us to frame an initial inquiry into the relation between individual psychic structure and its surrounding field or group context. They tend, however, to conceptualize fields and groups in terms of regressive processes. Freud (1921) described, in group formation, a "dwindling of the conscious individual personality," a "focusing of thoughts and feelings into a common direction," a "predominance of the affective side of the mind and of unconscious psychical life," and a "tendency to the immediate carrying out of intentions as the emergey"—all of which corresponds to "a state of regression . . . of just such a sort as we should be inclined to ascribe to the primal horde" (p. 122). Bion (1961) elaborated that "in a group the adult resorts, in what may be a massive regression to mechanisms . . . typical of the earliest phases of mental life" (p. 141). The Barangers and Baranger (1964) write of analytic field as a 'regressive situation,' one of mutual projective identification, in which "the analyst is the analysand's 'adult,' 'healthy,' ego etc., and the analysand is the 'child,' the 'neurotic,' etc. who lies inside the analyst" (p. 11). These roles may, however, reverse, as they realize, such that the analyst becomes the 'sick child,' and the analysand is the 'healthy adult.'

Here the analyst or group leader is the mature one; the patient or group members are the childish ones. The roles may change temporarily. It is acknowledged, moreover, that the patient-as-child performs a container function for the analyst's projection of his own inner child. The basic division of roles presupposes, however, a normative hierarchy of maturity. The hierarchy of field maturity re-inscribes, on an interpersonal level, the problems of regression already discussed: the genetic fallacy, the morality of maturity, etc.

Pre-Oedipal Dependency

A related but separate trend in pre-Oedipal research highlights the importance of the early relational environment in the development of psychic structure (Hartmann, 1939; Winnicott, 1954a, 1954b; Balint, 1968; Mahler, 1975; Kohut, 1971). Dependency needs, for example, to be held, soothed, or mirrored, are considered to be uniquely infantile in nature. The persistence of intense dependency longings, manifest in the transference, is framed, accordingly, as a sign of deficit and arrest at a pre-Oedipal phase of mental development.

The pre-Oedipal slant, however, sets up a tautology (see Chapter 2). It has become a commonplace that the person (healthy or ill) is inextricably embedded in interpersonal dependencies. What was once considered a fact of pre-Oedipal development and, tautologically, a sign of a universal regressive striving, is now recognized an existential fact of life across the lifespan. If we consider intense dependency a unique feature of childhood (not just a fact of life), then, when we inevitably discover the adult patient's profound dependencies, it will seem evidence of a regressive trend. To get beyond the prejudice, we must acknowledge not only childhood dependency but normative adult dependency.

The Relational Matrix

The pursuit of a non-regressive field theory leads into interpersonal-relational and intersubjective theories of the relational matrices in which we remain embedded across the lifespan. Sullivan wrote little about field per se. The idea of the field was, however, essential in his thinking (Stern, 2015). In two of his more explicit descriptions, he wrote that

> Scientific psychiatry has to be defined as the study of interpersonal relations, and this in the end calls for the use of the kind of conceptual framework that we now call *field theory* [sic]. From such a standpoint, personality is taken to be hypothetical. That which can be studied is the pattern of processes which characterize the interaction of personalities in particular recurrent situations or fields which 'include' the observer. Since any one participant observer can study but a finite number of these situations or fields, which, in turn, will be anything but representative of the whole variegated world of human life, not all of the personality of the observer will be revealed and 'what he comes to know about himself' will always be somewhat incomplete and variously contingent. . . . Generalizations which he can make about 'the other fellow' cannot but be even more incomplete and contingent.
>
> (Sullivan, 1953, p. 368)

And later,

> Every constructive effort of the psychiatrist, today, is a strategy of interpersonal field operations which (1) seek to map the areas of disjunctive force that block the efficient collaboration of the patient and others, and (2) seeks to expand the patient's awareness so that this unnecessary blockage can be brought to an end.
>
> (Sullivan, 1953, p. 376)

The field, in Sullivan's usage, is the interpersonal situation. The person does not exist outside of it. Even when he is alone, as Stern (2015) elaborates, the person is a product of past and present fields. The field shapes his most private unconscious desires and fantasies. It also determines what cannot be thought. The therapist helps the patient by mapping interpersonal blockages and, through insight, facilitating greater interpersonal freedom.

Sullivan (1953) recognized that, as a person with his own interpersonal distortions, the therapist would have his own blockages or limitations in facilitating this inquiry. "It must be noted," He wrote, "that an identical distortion of living common to doctor and patient makes this type of inquiry, at best, very difficult" (p. 377). The therapist should strive, albeit as an unattainable ideal, to integrate his dissociated interpersonal patterns, so that he can take his own field involvement into account. "We can improve our techniques for participant observation in an interpersonal situation in which we are integrated with our subject-person. This is evidently *the* procedure of psychiatry" (p. 5).

Later interpersonal-relational theorists questioned the tenability of this ideal. "It began to be understood," Stern (2015) writes, "that the analyst was involved with the patient in a way that, while maintaining the behavioral and experiential reciprocity Sullivan describes, did not necessarily allow the analyst's consistent, conscious observation of this reciprocal involvement" (p. 39). The analyst's expertise was re-defined accordingly. It no longer implied a superior awareness of the significance of one's conduct, but rather a capacity to engage analytically in non-transparent field situations.

Levenson (1972), an early proponent of this shift in thinking, argued that "perhaps the single most significant observation for therapy, whatever the content of the session, it will simultaneously be played out, *choreographed* in the metacommunication of therapist and patient" (pp. 188–189.). In short, "the formal aspects of the session replicate the content." The therapist becomes an unwitting actor in the co-created drama. Stern (2005) elaborates, in a new introduction to Levenson's book, that, "without realizing it, the analyst of a masochistic patient makes sadistic interpretations of masochism; the analyst of a seductive patient makes seductive interpretations of the patient's fear; the analyst of a narcissistically vulnerable patient interprets the narcissism in a way that wounds" (p. vii). The ideal therapist is, Levenson holds, willing to 'trip' with the patient, and, through awareness, to resist unreflective assimilation into the transactional field (p. 214). The assimilation, however, with or without insight, is inevitable and continuous. Today's insight disrupts a transactional pattern *and* is already part of a new one.

Relational psychoanalysis—a collection of integrative perspectives, which, like the British Independent School, encompasses a set of related but different viewpoints—developed in America in an explicit effort to bring interpersonal psychoanalysis, object relations, self-psychology, and aspects of contemporary Freudian thought into a common dialogue. Perhaps the most salient defining feature of this group is its rejection of drive theory in favor of a metapsychological stance in which the self–other relationship, not discharge per se, is the primary object of study (Mitchell & Greenberg, 1983; Mitchell, 1988). The term *relationship* carries the dual sense here of intrapsychic and interpersonal relations.

The relational matrix—the here-and-now field of intrapsychic and interpersonal configurations—is the focal point, in relational thought, of theoretical integration and clinical inquiry (Mitchell, 1988). "The most useful way to view psychological reality," Mitchell writes, "is as operating within a relational matrix which encompasses both intrapsychic and interpersonal realms" (p. 9). The concept of the relational matrix implies the notion of a relational unconscious analogous to unconscious group phantasy life in Bion. An emergent phenomenon, it operates as an 'unrecognized bond' of mutual influence between participants (Gerson, 2004). It exists only within the interpersonal situation (broadly construed to include periods of physical distance between the participants).

Some relationalists believe that, to take account of our immersion in relational matrices, out of which all lived experience is co-created, we must transition from a repression model to a dissociation model of the mind (Davies, 1996; Stern, 2003b, 2015). Davies (1996), for instance, argues against the idea of a dynamic unconscious comprised of fixed repressed ideas or memories. She proposes a relational model in which there is no stable or consistent repression barrier. Rather, "what is conscious or unconscious . . . will emerge fluidly out of the particular constellation of self and object-related experience that crystallizes in the foreground of interpersonal experience at any given moment" (p. 562). Certain self-states are, in this model, felt to be incompatible and are therefore held in dissociation, instead of being repressed. That is to say, they are lived, and sometimes consciously recognized, but independently, rigidly, without creative interplay. The subject proves unable to "stand in the spaces" (Bromberg, 1996) between them.

Stern (2003b, 2015) gives dissociation a more radical meaning. For him, dissociation refers not to the segregation of formulated self-states, but to a more severe defense in which the person does not formulate or represent painful experience. This becomes 'unformulated experience,' a term that overlaps with Bion's notion of beta-elements. We encounter the unformulated, in a parallel with the Kleinian/Bionian tradition, through interpersonal enactment: "the attribution of one's dissociated parts to the other, who one then treats as the alien, dissociated part of oneself" (Stern, 2015, p. 111).

Field shifts enable the emergence and formulation the unformulated. The shifts themselves are mysterious and beyond operationalization.

> We want to do whatever is possible to become aware of, and then loosen, constricted interaction, thereby promoting therapeutic action by unlocking the capacity of relatedness to serve as the crucible for the unbidden. But because these events—this relaxation of relatedness—are and *emergent* [sic] quality of the relatedness itself, it is impossible to specify in advance a technique to accomplish it.
>
> (p. 115)

Here we find a difference between the relational and the Bionian traditions, as developed, for instance, in Ferro's work, in that the former puts greater emphasis on implicit relational shifts, which enable insight, while the latter puts greater emphasis on interpretations, albeit 'weak' ones, which help transform beta into alpha-elements.

The latter difference in emphasis can lead, however, to a false dichotomy. In the interpersonal-relational tradition, Stern writes, "the emphasis falls on the mutative effects of freeing clinical relatedness," while, in more traditional approaches, the emphasis falls on the interpretive understanding of transference (p. 114). But the difference in emphasis "should not obscure the recognition that analysts of all persuasions work and think in both ways." Perhaps transference interpretation is best conceived as a kind of relational move. If one adopts this stance, it would become a category error to pit the one against the other.

The dissociation movement puts a strong emphasis on the here-and-now co-creation of experience. But it depends, in my reading, on too narrow a view of repression—a definition that, in turn, makes it easy to reject repression model of the unconscious. According to this view, repression is a defense by which fixed ideas and memories are kept unconscious. The basic claim is that, since no mental content is fixed, and everything exists in the field-contingent flux of formulation/non-formulation, the very idea of a stable repression barrier, keeping down set content, is phenomenologically inapt.

I contend, by contrast, that the repressed is not fixed, but like the dissociated, field-contingent. Melanie Klein (1959) suggested a similar view in her contention that, "whenever we can admire and love somebody—or hate and despise somebody—we also take something of them into ourselves and our deepest attitudes are shaped by such experiences" (p. 256). The person unconsciously condenses (Freud, 1915) new field experiences into repressed ideas, affects and memories, which, are, in turn, reshaped by them.

The result is a more conservative relational view in which repression and dissociation are both available. We already find such an integration in Bromberg (1996), who holds that, even in health, a "normal personality structure is shaped by dissociation as well as by repression" (p. 512). One form of dissociation keeps apart subjectively incompatible self-states. A more severe, but equally common, form of dissociation prevents painful states from being formulated/represented. Repression buries conflictual-formulated, but fluid and field-contingent, experience within the immediate relational matrix.

The Intersubjective Tradition

A third tradition, which intersects conceptually with Bionian and relational field theory, albeit with little cross-referencing between groups, derives from Kohut and finds its fullest expression in Stolorow, Atwood, Brandchaft and Orange's intersubjective approach.

The concept of the selfobject (Kohut, 1971, 1977, 1984) is a field concept without an explicit field theory. Kohut (1971) introduced the term in a departure from the position, exemplified in Freud's (1914) paper on narcissism, that there is a dialectical tension between narcissism, on the one hand, and, on the other hand, investment in object relations. He introduced the term selfobject to refer to various modes of narcissistic object investment, a term which, by definition, dissolves the dichotomy between self and object-cathexis:

> One of the difficulties encountered as one approaches the theoretical problems of narcissism . . . is the frequently made assumption that the existence of object relations excludes narcissism. On the contrary . . . some of the most intense narcissistic experiences relate to objects: objects, that is, which are either used in the service of the self and of the maintenance of its instinctual investment, or objects which are themselves experienced as part of the self. I shall refer to the latter as *selfobjects* [sic].
>
> (Kohut, 1971, p. xiv.)

The person invests in the self through the object in the partial merger experience of the selfobject. He does not, as in Freud's theory of primary narcissism, cathect the ego before the object. Nor does he retreat, as in Freud's theory of secondary narcissism, from the object into an ego cathexis. Here the person's self-investment always includes the object tie.

Kohut (1971, 1977) and his students (cf. Terman, 1984; Wolf, 1988; Stolorow, Atwood, & Brandchaft, 1992) elaborated various modes self-object relating, with an initial emphasis on pre-Oedipal development and a gradual expansion to cover the entire lifespan. Kohut's (1971) early formulation highlighted three forms of mirroring, manifest in pre-Oedipal development, later revived in the analytic situation in form of the mirror transference: merger (in which the object is experienced as an extension of the grandiose self, like a body part, with analogous expectations of unquestioned dominance), twinship (in which the object is experienced as being like the grandiose self in psychological makeup), and mirroring in the narrow sense (in which the object is experienced as a separate entity, but is important to the subject, and is accepted by him, only as a source of affirmation). Kohut (1977), Terman (1984) and Wolf (1988) extended the self-object concept to capture the self-affirming quality of healthy Oedipal object relations, for example, the mother's prideful response to her son's budding sense of masculinity, complimented, in optimal development, by the non-defensive father's playful acceptance of his adversarial role. On a more fundamental level, operative before and continuous with the above selfobject modes, Stolorow, Atwood and Brandchaft (1992), by contrast, have posited a self-delineating selfobject function: the other's function in helping the child (or adult) to articulate his inner experience, organizing his subjective reality, and strengthening his confidence in its validity.

The concept of the intersubjective field originates, in this tradition, its many other psychoanalytic and philosophical influences notwithstanding, in a universalization of the selfobject concept. "The conceptualization of an intersubjective field is, in part," Stolorow and Atwood (1984) write, "an attempt to lift the selfobject concept to a higher, more inclusive level of generality" (p. 54). Every phase of development—not just the earliest phases—are conceptualized, in this model, in terms of the "psychological field constituted by the intersection of the child's evolving subjective universe with those of caretakers" (p. 55). Self-object transference is no longer a *kind* of transference. Rather, it is, in this extension, a "dimension of all transference, which may fluctuate in the extent to which it occupies a position of figure or ground" (Stolorow, Brandchaft, & Atwood, 1987, p. 41.)

The authors build on this foundation to develop a critique of temporal regression, while maintaining the possibility of structural regression. "No doubt archaic modes of psychological organization in adults are related to the psychological organizations found in childhood," write Stolorow, Brandchaft and Atwood (1987)."However, these archaic modes are not identical with their manifestations and occurrences in the young child" (p. 30). The implication is that 'archaic' mentation develops from its infantile to its adult manifestations. The ever-changing field ensures, even in the most stubborn repetitions, a degree of novelty in the form, content and function of one's desires, phantasies, defenses etc. To admit this critique, while retaining structural regression, the authors restrict the latter to designate shifts from more mature to more archaic levels of psychological organization. It is essential that, since the adult-archaic ≠ the infantile-archaic, a structural regression does not, for these authors, imply a temporal regression to earlier forms.

The unconscious is organized, in this vision of the present adult field, into three realms (Stolorow, Atwood, & Brandchaft, 1992). The 'dynamic unconscious' refers to repressed (but at least partially formulated/symbolized) memories, fantasies, feelings and other experiential content. The 'prereflective unconscious' consists of the organizing principles by which the person shapes and thematizes his experience. The 'unvalidated unconscious' consists of experiences that were never articulated (not even partially) because they did not evoke the requisite validating response from the surround. If the dynamic unconscious content lies in the figurative basement of the mind-as-building, and the pre-reflective unconscious refers to the architect's blueprints, then the unvalidated unconscious refers to the "bricks, lumber and other unused materials left lying around the building," materials that could be made part of the construction, but have been left in disarray (p. 35).

Like Bromberg (1996), then, the intersubjectivists posit an unconscious in which we find both repressed representations and unrepresented experience. There is no need, in this theory, to choose between a model of repressed contents and one of unrepresented experience.

Perhaps the greatest difficulty, if we are to put intersubjective field tradition in dialogue with the other major field traditions, lies in the former's repudiation of the concept of projective identification. The concept, according to Stolorow, Orange and Atwood's (1998, 2001) critique, allows the analyst to transform his disruptive visceral experiences, and his emergent fantasy of being invaded by the patient, into a linear cause-effect reality: The patient's projection is thought to *cause* the analyst's state. The authors hold that, in this act of reification, the analyst constructs a demonology with no real explanatory power, but, on the negative side, a great risk of imposing one's fantasy on the patient, who, it is feared, must either agree compliantly, or risk making the analyst feel impotent. Behind this error are the workings of a one-person psychology, which, the authors hold, is unable to account for the nonlinear dynamic emergence of the states in question.

Stolorow, Orange and Atwood (1998) conclude that Kleinian theory, including its interpersonalized offshoots (e.g., Bionian field theory) and intersubjectivity theory are "incommensurable paradigms," with "no metaphors, no vocabulary, and no conception of human nature and of human possibility in common" (p. 723). To the extent that some relational theorists continue to use the concept of projective identification (e.g., Ogden, 1982; Stern, 1994; Aron, 1996), Stolorow, Orange and Atwood consider them to be mired in the discourse of a one-person psychology incapable of realizing our full intersubjective embeddedness.

There is, however, a potential opening for integration, the difficulties notwithstanding, in Ogden's (1982) reformulation of projective identification, which can support a revised Bionian group theory (Rizzolo, 2012) and, in turn, a more compatible Bionian field theory. In Bion's (1961) version of projective identification, the container's personality is obliterated. His model *is* a one-person psychology in so far as the container makes no subjective contribution to the co-creation of the contained. In Ogden's version, by contrast, we find a three-step process: (1) The projector phantasizes that he has put a part of himself in the recipient; (2) the projector behaves in such a way as to coerce the recipient into compliance with the projection; (3) the recipient, who responds out of his own subjectivity, phantasizes that he does, in fact, contain something that the patient has projected. The result is a co-created phantasy with subjective contributions from both participants.

It is unclear why such an interaction, of all potential interactions, could not occur in intersubjective field theory. It would seem that the two field participants could have any shared fantasy imaginable—including the shared fantasy specified by the concept of projective identification. The intersubjectivists' main point, as I understand it, is that such a process is nonlinear: the projector does not cause or determine the analyst's feeling state any more than the analyst causes or determines the projector's projected content. The two are embedded in a field, which is comprised by the intersection of their subjectivities, prior to the emergence of private or shared phantasies of projection and introjection. In other words, the projected has already been co-constructed prior to projection.

Nachträglichkeit

The co-creation of experience and meaning, on conscious and unconscious levels, occurs in a relational field. The key point for my argument—one with which few would disagree—is that the subjects in a field co-create meaning irreducible to any historical precursor. We must recognize the *historicity of experience* amidst the emergence of *new forms*.

The co-constructive process occurs in two ways. It involves, on the one hand, as we have seen, the co-creation of previously unformulated or unthinkable thoughts and affects. It involves, on the other hand, the re-configuration of historically embedded thoughts, feelings, memories, needs, wishes and internal representations in emergent ways.

The two aspects of this process can be understood in terms of a broadened conception of *Nachträglichkeit*, or 'deferred action,' which, in this approach, becomes a universal principle of development. The concept of *Nachträglichkeit* captures the idea that

> experiences, impressions and memory traces may be revised at a later date to fit with fresh experiences or with the attainment of a new stage of development. They may in that event be endowed not only with a new meaning but with psychical effectiveness.
>
> (Laplanche & Pontalis, 1973, p. 110)

The result is a cyclical, rather than a linear, view of psychic determinism. The past acts upon the present. And the present conditions the past. The present does not change actual history, but it alters, through selective attention, and through the retroactive ascription of meaning to old experiences, which thereby gain new efficacy, the past's residue in the unconscious.

The idea stems from a series of scattered, but suggestive, comments throughout Freud's writing. 'Memory,' he wrote, in one of the clearest early articulations of the idea, "is present not once, but several times over. . . . It is laid down in various kinds of indications. . . . The successive registrations represent the psychic achievement of successive epochs of life" (Masson, 1985, p. 207). We find a concrete example in the case of the Wolf Man (Freud, 1918). The Wolf Man, according to Freud, witnessed the primal scene at 18 months. He first took it to be a violent act. Later at age 4, he dreamt of wolves outside his window. The dream, Freud interpreted, represented his wish to occupy his mother's position in what he retrospectively understood to be an act of pleasure. In light of subsequent castration threats, his passive sexual wish amounted to castration. Only then—after the deferred action of the dream—did he develop a wolf phobia.

The Freudian notion of deferred action pertains narrowly to experiences that have been repressed: "It is not lived experience in general that undergoes a deferred revision but, specifically, whatever it has been impossible in the first instance to incorporate fully into a meaningful context" (Laplanche & Pontalis, 1973, p. 111). More recent theorists do, however, broaden the term. For Modell (1990), it becomes a general principle of development. "If we put aside the specific issue of sexual trauma," Modell (1990) writes, "the principle that Freud proposed is: *the ego can constantly remodel memory in accordance with current and immediate experience* [*sic*]" (1990, p. 17). All memory is, he argues, a form of re-categorization in which old categories are re-imagined in light of new experience. Our deepest memory traces evolve, on a neurological level, such that their record in the central nervous system is no longer isomorphic with the original memory trace (Modell, 1990; Edelman, 1987). Here *Nachträglichkeit*, or 'retranscription,' in Model's terms, is not an isolated event, but a process at play in all mentation.

The term *retranscription* presupposes a first transcription. Faimberg (2007), who also supports a broadened use of *Nachträglichkeit*, adds that deferred action sometimes gives a first meaning, or transcription, to the unformulated. She outlines a two-phase developmental sequence. First, in the *anticipation* phase, the subject registers a 'presentation' without a meaning. In the second phase, which she terms the *assignment of retroactive meaning*, the subject gives the anticipatory presentation it's first-ever construction. It leads, then, from an initial unrepresented impression into a first-time understanding.

This two-phase process is reminiscent, albeit with a special emphasis on the retrospective gaze, of the transformation of beta into alpha-elements

(Bion), the co-creation of the unformulated (Stern), and the validation of the unvalidated (Stolorow and Atwood). It indicates the possibility of extending the concept of *Nachträglichkeit* beyond repressed (formulated) memories to the realm of unformulated perceptions and proto-emotions.

I use the term *deferred action* in its broadened sense. The broadened term rules out the possibility of unaltered unconscious infantile mentation. Even the earliest needs wishes, thoughts and feelings develop via retranscription and, in some cases, first-time transcription. It follows that the unconscious—at all levels of depth—does develop over time. The work of deferred action results, through each phase of life, in an effective personal history: a history of lifespan effects embedded in the unconscious (Rizzolo, 2016).

The return of a childhood memory, desire, phantasy or defense is often termed a regression. But, if we accept a generalized model of deferred action, then it is never a true return. It is, rather, a progression into the re-constellation of the familiar in a novel form.

The Kleinian Marriage: An Illustration

The concept of *Nachtraglichkeit* can help us, for example, to understand Melanie Klein's (1937) account of internal growth in a stable and satisfactory love relationship in adulthood:

> A relationship of this nature affords the widest scope for the most varied manifestations of love. If the woman has a maternal attitude towards the man, she satisfies (as far as can be) his earliest wishes for the gratifications he desired from his own mother. In the past, these wishes have never been quite satisfied, and have never been quite given up. The man has now, as it were, this mother for his own, with relatively little feeling of guilt. . . . If the woman has a richly developed emotional life, besides possessing these maternal feelings, she will also have kept something of the child's attitude towards her father, and some of the features of this old relationship will enter into her relation to her husband; for instance, she will trust and admire her husband, and he will be a protective and helpful figure to her as her father was. These feelings will be a foundation for a relation in which the woman's desires and needs as a grown-up person can find full satisfaction. Again, this attitude of his wife's gives the man the

> opportunity to be protective and helpful to her in various ways—that is, in his unconscious mind, to play the part of a good husband to his mother.
>
> (p. 313)

The man finds, in his wife, a nurturing maternal presence; and the woman finds, in him, a protective and helpful father-figure. The interplay of past and present has mutual psychic effects. It changes each partner's unconscious sense of self in relation to his or her internal parents.

It tempers, for one, the woman's early hostility toward her parents and thereby strengthens her confidence in their durable internal presence and in her own restorative capacities:

> I have mentioned before the importance of the little girl's unconscious wish to receive a baby from her father, and of the sexual desires towards him which are connected with this wish. The father's frustration of her genital desires gives rise to intense aggressive phantasies in the child. . . . In her jealousy and hatred she wishes it to be a dangerous and evil thing—one which could not gratify her mother either—and the penis thus, in her phantasy, acquires destructive qualities. . . . The aggressive phantasies are again followed in the child's mind by wishes to make good—more specifically, by phantasies of healing the father's genital which, in her mind, she has injured or made bad.
>
> (p. 314)

If in adulthood her husband

> Loves her and also gratifies her sexually, her unconscious sadistic phantasies will lose in strength. But since these are not entirely put out of action . . . they lead to a stimulation of phantasies of a restoring nature; thus once more the drive to make reparation is brought into action . . . because there is somewhere in the depths of her mind a feeling that her genital is dangerous and could injure her husband's genital—which is a derivative of her aggressive phantasies towards her father—one part of the satisfaction she obtains comes from the fact that she is capable of giving her husband pleasure and happiness, and that her genital thus proves to be good . . . [and] if she has a happy

> and sexually gratifying relationship with her husband, his genital is felt to be good, and thus her fears of the bad genital are disproved. The sexual gratification thus works as a double reassurance: of her own goodness and of her husband's.
>
> (p. 314)

She finds reassurance, through their mutually satisfying relationship, that

> Her sadistic wishes against her mother have not taken effect, or that reparation has succeeded. . . . she is [now] able to feel equal to her mother, to enjoy the same happiness, rights and privileges as her mother did, but without injuring and robbing her.
>
> (pp. 315–316)

The adult love relationship thus modifies her aggression and reassures her of her own goodness. She gains an improved relationship with her internal parents. It does not alter their historical reality but perhaps makes newly available benign qualities once lost in her hostility.

The man, for his part, finds a similar reassurance in his wife's love and appreciation. The relationship, if it is a satisfying one, softens early sadistic impulses, repairs the bond with his internal parents and brings a newfound confidence in his own goodness:

> The frustration by his mother of his genital desires in his childhood aroused phantasies in which his penis became an instrument which could give pain and cause injury to her. At the same time jealousy and hatred of his father as a rival for his mother's love set going phantasies of a sadistic nature against his father also.
>
> (p. 315)

If in adulthood he can satisfy his wife,

> the penis is then felt to be a good and curative organ, which shall afford the woman pleasure, cure her injured genital and create babies in her. A happy and sexually gratifying relationship with the woman affords him proofs of the goodness of his penis, and also unconsciously gives him the feeling that his wishes to restore her have succeeded.
>
> (p. 315)

Not only does their love repair his relation to his internal mother, but it

> has also the effect of diminishing his aggression against his father, which was greatly stimulated by his being unable to have his mother as a wife, and this may reassure him that his long-standing sadistic tendencies against his father have not been effective. . . . To possess his wife's love and appreciation gives him a feeling of being fully grown-up and thus of being equal to his father. The hostile and aggressive rivalry with him diminishes and gives way to a more friendly competition with his father—or rather with admired father figures—in productive functions and achievements, and this is very likely to enhance or increase his productivity.
>
> (pp. 315–316)

Like his wife, the husband find his sadism lowered, and his good, restorative capacities affirmed. He thereby gains an improved relationship with his internal parents. He is better able to forgive the frustrations at his mother's hands and to regard his father, with a new sense of equality, and thus with less hatred and jealousy, as a friendly and admired rival.

The mutual love of man and woman initiates a retranscription of their internal parents. The retranscription, which can be considered a deferred action, makes available benign and restorative aspects of the internal self-parent bond before extant only as latent potential. The improved internal relationship can, in turn, feedback into the adult love relationship. The result is a generative cycle of *Nachtraglichkeit*. It is implied that a hostile adult love relationship would result in the opposite: a vicious cycle of deferred action.

The adult relationship illustrates how the here-and-now intersubjective field can initiate a process a deferred action by which the efficacy of past events is modified and developed. If we take this illustration not as unique to adult love, but as representative of people grow and change, at all levels of depth, through their present relationships, across the lifespan, it would seem that that the analytic relationship, too, can have such deferred effects.

The analytic field, it then follows, modifies the object of its own inquiry prior to interpretation.[1] It modifies repressed contents, for example, through softening or exacerbating the hostility of latent self and object representations, before they manifest in play or speech. It complicates pre-reflective organizing principles, for example, the subject's way of dealing with the mother's seductiveness or the father's counter-aggression, by integrating them with the emergent, but still implicit, ways of dealing with the analyst's seductiveness or hostility. It opens and, at the same time, limits the new sphere of what can and cannot be formulated, for example, how one might recognize—even unconsciously—if it is to be recognized at all—that the analyst seems, like the father, to be jealous of the subject's anticipated successes. The work of analysis appears, in this reading, to be the analysis of deferred action.

Child and Adolescent Characters

Ferro (1999, 2002) imagines the psychoanalytic session as being populated with 'characters' (e.g., the characters of an anecdote, a memory, a story or a dream). These are sometimes, as Spillius (1999) clarifies, 'personifications' in the patient's or analyst's material. They can also be mental processes (e.g. "a memory as a character" Ferro, 1999b, p. 95).

The characters of a session, unlike those in a text, lack a pre-established narrative fate. The analytic couple re-imagines the former continuously through projection and dialogue:

> Whereas a literary character is not only a construction present in the narration and endowed with an essential structure of its own, but also a reconstruction by the reader whereby it so to speak becomes actual instead of just potential, the psychoanalytic character lacks a given, objective aspect, because it is articulated progressively by way of the dialogic and projective interaction of patient and analyst: it is a dynamic entity that is never completely defined, of twofold paternity, subject to constant additions and modifications, with a double genetic heritage in a state of constant flux.
>
> (Ferro, 1999b, p. 90)

The psychoanalytic character, then, is co-authored from the beginning (and continuously re-imagined) through bi-directional projective and introjective exchanges, or as the intersubjectivists and some relationalists might prefer, through prereflective or implicit enactments. The original co-authorship sets him apart from the literary character, who already has a textual status, and is secondarily reconstructed or actualized in the reader's mind.

The analyst can listen and interpret the characters of a session, according to Ferro (1999a), with a hermeneutic interest in one or more of three end points: the patient's actual history (associated with Freud), the phantasies of the internal world (associated with Klein), or the functioning of the present field (associated with Bion and Ferro's own contribution). The characters of the session are, in the first hermeneutic, understood as the representations of actual historical people. The interpretive task is to trace the character back to the historical person or persons who are being represented. The characters are, in the second hermeneutic, understood as the representations of internal objects. The interpretive task is to identify the internal objects to which the characters correspond. The characters are, in the third hermeneutic, irreducible to real historical persons or pre-given internal objects. They are, though partly derivative of these influences, open to new constructions, not given in advance, but emergent in the context of the field. The interpretive task, in the third case, is not to find correlations (with actual historical people or with pre-given internal objects), but to be open to potential worlds of narration.

It sometimes happens that the character of the session is a young child or adolescent. The analyst might look for correlations between the young character and the patient's actual history (Ferro's first hermeneutic) or internal objects (Ferro's second hermeneutic). He might, in the first case, interpret that the character represents an actual early version of the patient. He might, in the second, interpret that the character represents an internal child—often with the assumption that it is an enduring relic of infantile phantasy life. These claims are often plausible and can serve pragmatic clinical purposes: the recovery of repressed memories and the integration of internal objects into the fabric of psychic life. The critique of regression would simply caution against correlations that are too strongly stated and/or unverifiable outside of theoretical pre-suppositions.

The young character can also, however, be seen as an emergent construct of the present field. It reflects not as an actual regression, then, but a special case of deferred action. It is the retroactive development and bringing into fruition of a potential that was only partly latent in the patient's history and in the network of internal objects already established. This development requires the field interaction for its actualization in the present. It is assumed that, if the field were different, the material might have developed differently. The task is not to correlate the emergent character with and pre-existing structure but rather, to entertain an openness to its nascent meaning and function in the field.

An example of this process can be found in Davies and Frawley's (1991) discussion of the 'child persona' in psychoanalytic work with the adult survivor of childhood sexual trauma. Their listening perspective in the following passages illustrates the first and second hermeneutics. They emphasize, to begin, that the child persona is not a metaphorical representation, but a 'concrete' structure with a 'primitive' system of defenses.

> It is remarkable to observe the degree to which most survivors can painstakingly erect the semblance of a functioning, adaptive, interpersonally related self around the screaming core of a wounded and abandoned child. . . . The patient who was sexually abused as a child is not an adult patient with particularly vivid memories of painful childhood experiences existing in the context of other, happier, more loving times. We stress here that this child is a fully developed, dissociated, rather primitively organized alternative self. In this regard we speak concretely, not metaphorically. It is imperative that the therapist who begins working with an adult who has survived significant childhood sexual abuse understand that he or she is, in fact, undertaking the treatment of two people: an adult who struggles to succeed, relate, gain acceptance, and ultimately to forget and a child who, as treatment progresses, strives to remember and to find a voice with which to scream out his or her outrage at the world.
>
> (p. 281)

By a 'dissociated,' 'primitively organized' self, the authors mean, more specifically, that dissociation

> preserves and protects, in split-off form, the entire internal object world of the abused child.
>
> (p. 274)

The persona often manifests in session with

> a different wardrobe, facial expressions, body postures, voice quality, and set of linguistic expressions. 'She' takes on the persona of a timid

> little girl; 'he,' of an awkward preadolescent whose emergent sexuality has lagged behind that of his chums.
>
> (p. 281)

From a developmental perspective,

> the child aspect of the self representation, along with that of the abusing other and their complex system of emotional connection and exchange, is cordoned off and isolated from the rest of the personality. It remains virtually frozen in time, the images unmodulated by any others of a different, perhaps gentler nature. . . . The child cannot grow. Her anger and self-hatred go untampered, therefore unintegrated. Her world is a world of betrayal, terror, and continued emotional flooding.
>
> (p. 286)

While the analyst and the patient's adult-self interview develop a relationship, the child-self

> is kept very far away from the analytic field. The child has little or no impact on the analytic relationship, and this relationship has affected her only insofar as she has perceived enough trust between the analyst and the adult to encourage her participation.
>
> (p. 285)

The adult's child persona, in this understanding, is a literal (not metaphorical) psychic structure. It is held to preserve, in an unaltered form, the internal object world of the actual abused child. It exists, the authors hold, almost entirely outside of the analytic field. When it does emerge in the session, in speech or nonverbal action, it can be correlated, in the first and second hermeneutics, with the real past and the frozen internal world.

The analytic task, in this model, is to make contact with the dissociated child persona within the abused adult, which, through projection and introjection, enters the therapeutic relationship, where it can be interpreted, enabling a resumption of growth and integration. The question, from the vantage point of the third hermeneutic, is whether the child persona is, in fact, outside of the field, or whether it is reconfigured, by immersion in the field (implicit in the act of projection/introjection) prior to verbal interpretation or integration. In other words: How might the analytic field modify that which has remained frozen—for example, preserving the intensity of the rage and shame—but shifting the contours of the ice?

The clinical picture in Frawley and Davies' paper suggests that the subject does update the child persona, even though it remains dissociated, in the surround of the present field. The child persona evolves, for example, through its interaction with the adult-persona. A frequent result is a complication of the original trauma with feelings of self-betrayal:

> Although the adult and the child are, in most situations, aware of each other, they are not friends. They have entirely different emotional agendas and live in a constant state of warfare over whose needs will take priority at any given time. Each feels entirely abandoned by the other. The child believes that the adult has 'sold out' by progressing with her life as a grown-up. After all, grown-ups are bad and do bad things. To become one of them is the ultimate betrayal.
>
> (p. 282)

The actual child dealt with the original trauma at the hands of an adult abuser. The child persona within the adult must now confront the additional betrayal of her own adult-persona. This complication of the trauma in the present field of development reshapes the ice.

The child persona retaliates against the adult-persona by attempting to subvert her growth. The reversal of abuser-abused roles is another development in the inner child's history:

> [The child self] uses the techniques she was taught by her abusive parent (other) to undermine the confidence of her other self: seduction, cajoling manipulation, and threat of abuse (in this case self-inflicted). As she herself felt invaded, she often invades the unexpecting, conscious sensorium of the adult in inappropriate and disruptive ways, causing great confusion and disorientation, at times bringing to a halt whatever activity the adult was engaged in at that moment. She stands in relation to her adult-self—a provocateur, with a terrorists commitment to a program of unrelenting insurgence.
>
> (p. 282)

The child-self thus transforms into a provocateur that was not part of the original child's experience. It is an intrapsychic complication of a kind that can occur only after the subject has matured and finds, in her nascent adult self, a betrayal in the form of growing up.

The adult-persona, in return, hates the disruptive child-self and blames her for the original abuse in a reinforcement, with new ammunition, of any original self-blame in childhood. This is another development in the cumulative trauma suffered by adult survivor:

> On her end, the adult persona 'hates' the sadistic and disruptive child with bitter intensity. On the most conscious level, the adult views the child as a demanding, entitled, rebellious and petulant pain in the neck. If she remembers being sexually abuse in childhood, she blames her child-self for the abuse and thereby refortifies her insistence on the child's thorough and complete badness.
>
> (p. 282)

The adult's hatred of the child persona and, more specifically, her inclination to blame the child persona for being abused, is exacerbated by the fact that, acting as her child-self, she is, as we have seen, guilty of initiating and propelling self-abusive patterns in the present. The reality of the child-persona's present culpability mixes with the (false) belief that she was responsible, as an actual child, for causing the original abuse she suffered. This mixture complicates whatever was the actual child's original feeling of self-blame and, for the adult in therapy, makes it all the harder to accept the child persona.

By 'frozen' or 'undeveloped,' Frawley and Davies mean that the subject's original terror, shame, anger, guilt and self-hatred—and the relevant self and object representations—go untempered and therefore remain unintegrated with the maturing personality. The above reading suggests that, while this is true, development, in the sense of a progressive complication, does happen. The complication unfolds through deferred action: The efficacy of the early trauma is elaborated through subsequent events of the lifespan.

The process of deferred action continues within the analytic field, modifying the patient's dissociated self-structure, prior to explicit verbal interpretation, through ongoing enactment. In one such enactment we find a complimentary interaction between the patient's long held phantasy of being cared for and protected by an 'omnipotent rescuer' and the analyst's phantasy of being such a figure in the life of this 'frightened child' (pp. 290–291). The complimentary interaction begins with a therapist who, in listening to the patient's memories of terror and helplessness, is thrown back upon his own experiences of terror and helplessness, and, placing himself, his own children, or phantasied children in her situation, is moved to provide a quality of concern and support that she missed in childhood. The patient, who might initially require therapeutic adaptations, for example double sessions or phone-contact, is reassured, but also frightened, by the feeling that she has "found an ally at long last, someone who will listen, care and respect her particular needs for support, while she recovers and works through memories of her abuse" (p. 291). In his effort to adapt, the therapist inadvertently encourages the patient's phantasy that she will receive compensation for her abuse in the form of the therapist's concern and devotion. He thereby interferes with her mourning process. Her demands intensify, against the backdrop of her disappointment in the inefficacy of the therapist's care, with the inevitable result that the therapist, who is engaged in a masochistic surrender, will fail her.

The patient's disappointment re-activates her sadistic attitude toward her own dependency longings. Her sadism integrates her actual childhood hatred of her own longings, which she blames, in part, for causing her to seduce her abuser, with her adult hatred of her child persona, which, as we have seen, represents her ongoing dependency needs. She blames herself for letting herself being misled the therapist; and she blames the therapist, whom she now attempts to show up as false savior, for making empty promises.

The therapist, who experiences himself as a concerned and devoted listener, comes to regard the patient as a cruel, demanding, seductive, insatiable and dangerous abuser. What was once adaptation to need becomes a desperate eagerness to appease the other.

Frawley and Davies, who reject the ideal of the analyst as a 'dispassionate commentator,' assert that it is only by entering, via such enactments, the patient's dissociated world that he can understand the patient's experience of betrayal and distortion and, on this basis, make attuned interpretations that promote insight and integration. Their position is reminiscent of Levenson's belief (see above) that the therapist always becomes an unwitting actor in the co-created drama of the interpersonal field.

The question emerges, with Ferro's third hermeneutic in mind, of whether the child persona might be understood, in addition to being the representative of a literal psychic structure, and without denying its origins in a real abusive history, as a field character. Frawley and Davies suggest that, through her unreasonable demands and provocations, the patient unconsciously tests the analyst in hopes of discovering that the analyst, while flexible and supportive, is strong enough to establish reasonable limits and boundaries. The analyst's strength reassures her that "the analyst will be neither gobbled up by insatiable demands nor moved to a form of retaliation against the patient that could destroy the treatment" (p. 295). The failure to set limits, often coupled with unwitting retaliations against the patient, will, by contrast, confirm her fears and intensify feelings of rage, betrayal and futility. The implication is that the quality and intensity of the child-persona's affective state (e.g., her rage, terror, or sense of need) reflects, in addition to the residue of an actual childhood state, the ameliorative and/or iatrogenic functioning of the field.

The deferred action of the analytic field can exacerbate or temper the efficacy of the original trauma, represented by the dissociated child persona, such that the analysis ends in a tragic impasse, or, alternatively, such that the enactment can be contained and interpreted. The character of the child thus reflects the functioning of the patient–analyst couple. The enactment and interpretation go beyond the act of correlation (with real history or pre-set internal constellations) to the development of what is possible in the field

Note

1 Hoffman (1991, 1992) arrives at a similar point through the application of social constructivism to the psychoanalytic situation. The analyst and patient interact, he asserts, in conscious and unconscious ways to co-construct their experience. This is an ontological fact. The analyst cannot, through (illusory) efforts to master his countertransference, account for his influence fully and thereby achieve an impartial view of the patient.

Chapter 5

The Life Cycle (Without Regression)

The person, then, organizes his experience in a here-and-now field. If one considers the person's mental life as a whole, in the context of the immediate intersubjective milieu, then it becomes clear that artificially isolated motives, phantasies and defenses—whatever their origins—become part and parcel of a new organization in the present.

The relational and intersubjective theories of the field have, for the most part, emerged independently of the literature on lifespan development (Erikson, 1950; Galatzer-Levy & Cohler, 1993; Waddel, 1998). It is essential, however, to situate the field in the context of the lifespan. Without such an effort, psychoanalysis will tend, by default, to collapse the novel challenges of adulthood into the better theorized issues of childhood.

To move beyond regression models of development, one turns inevitably to lifespan accounts.[2] Current lifespan theories still rely, however, though to a diminishing degree, on the concept of regression (Erikson, 1950; Galatzer-Levy & Cohler, 1993; Waddell, 1998). They tend, more specifically, to posit an infantile unconscious that persists in the depths, and to which one can regress, through the subsequent phases of development. Without an alternative, it remains difficult to think about new development in depth: not as a superficial accretion, but as a deep modification of early intrapsychic structure.

The present chapter presents an irreversible lifespan narrative. It is a story in which one cannot regress. So-called regressions are themselves explored for new emergent qualities. The aim is to discern novelty in the re-iteration of early onset motives and patterns. The implication is that, by deconstructing regression logic, we can obtain a more accurate view of the adult patient. Instead of collapsing his issues into those of his early life, we can work to see how he has grown from childhood into a novel present.

I first review the previous argument to lay groundwork for an alternative lifespan account. Following an implicit suggestion in Erikson (1950), at which several later writers seem to have arrived independently, I propose that we can reframe regressions as shifts in the developmental present. The person shifts between positions in his struggle with persistent lifespan problems (Stern, 1985; Mitchell, 1988). To re-engage a lifespan problem is not to regress to the phase of its first manifestation. It is, on the contrary, to progress. Through deferred action, he progressively re-transcribes, and sometimes constitutes afresh, historically embedded wishes, feelings and memories (Modell, 1990; Faimberg, 2007). It is implicit that, as he develops, he mourns and reshapes the residues of a past now lost forever. To assert the irreversible nature of development is not to deny the importance of repetition. By re-transcribing old patterns in new contexts, the person produces emergent—though often familiar—self–other configurations (Galatzer-Levy, 2002). Novelty appears in the act of repetition. I explore a series of familiar 'regressions' from the psychoanalytic literature on development to discern the novelty at play.

The Critique of Regression

In the *Interpretation of Dreams* (1900), Freud introduced three interrelated forms of regression: formal (from conscious thoughts to primitive images and sensory traces), temporal (from later to earlier unconscious memories) and topographic (from the preconscious to the unconscious system). Shortly thereafter, he asserted that the libido could regress from psychic conflict to the erotogenic zones of earlier fixations (Freud, 1905). Later, he added that the ego could regress to earlier modes of functioning (Freud, 1917a).

Two overlapping traditions—a tradition of defensive regression and one of restorative regression—grew up around the basic premise that the subject can return to earlier phases of development (Rizzolo, 2016). The defensive tradition has focused historically on the defensive use of regression as an evasion of conflict (see, for example, Hartmann [1939] and Freud [1965] in ego psychology; see Klein [1946] and Fairbairn [1952] in object relations). The restorative tradition has focused on primary, that is, non-defensive, strivings to re-establish the merger conditions of the child–caregiver dyad (see, for example, Ferenczi's [1938] interpretation of Freud's libidinal stages; Balint [1959, 1968] and Winnicott [1954, 1955] in object relations; and Kohut [1971, 1977] in self-psychology).

Conservative critics of regression have endorsed the concept but qualified its usage. Arlow and Brenner (1964) argue, for instance, that regression is too often taken to implicate the entire psyche when, in fact, it impacts only certain functions within the apparatus. Other conservative critics argue that the psychoanalytic situation artificially induces the regression it observes in patients (Macalpine, 1950) and that psychoanalysts should not deliberately induce a regression beyond that with which the patient presents (Gill, 1984a).

A stronger critique emerges in the writing of Stolorow, Brandchaft, and Atwood (1987), Mitchell (1988), Wachtel (2008), and Inderbitzin and Levy (2000). These writers express concern about potential for what Erikson (1958) called 'originology' and Hartmann (1955) termed the 'genetic fallacy'—the tendency in psychoanalytic theory to reduce psychological experience and function in the present to its genetic origins in early life. The concept of regression enables the genetic fallacy by emphasizing the frequent likeness between past and present forms, while deemphasizing the differences. This, in turn, supports reductionist narratives of linear cause-effect from early fixation to present issue.

In previous chapters, I demonstrated that the stronger position relies on two propositions. First, psychoanalysis studies the person as an irreducible agent. It is epistemologically invalid to break him into regressive and mature parts. Second, psychoanalysis studies subjective meaning. The person always makes meaning in the present relational field. We must therefore seek the *present* meaning of childlike behavior.

In this chapter, I elaborate on the third and final proposition: that the person develops irreversibly through the lifespan. I go beyond current lifespan theories that still rely—through to a diminishing degree—on the term regression. The re-iteration of old behavior in a new phase is, by virtue of the new landscape, a new (non-regressive) event. What follows is, in one reviewer's words, a theory in which you can't go back home.

From Regressions to Shifts in Mental Organization

The concept of regression has, in fact, waned in its explanatory appeal among lifespan theorists. It has passed without much comment. In its place, we find a widespread interest in shifts in between mental states or positions amidst the complexities of the present field. I propose that we can salvage much of the clinical insight embedded in regression discourse by re-theorizing so-called regressions as shifts in the developmental present. The pay-off is increased attention to the novelty at play in new iterations of old patterns.

As early as Erikson (1950, 1958), we find a challenge to the conventional logic by which adults are reduced to psychological children. Psychoanalysis, he wrote, "has lifted to the rank of a cosmology the undeniable fact that man's adulthood contains a persistent childishness: that vistas of the future always reflect mirages of a missed past" (p. 18). The vistas of the future *do* reflect the mirages of the past. It is all too easy, however, to slip into 'originology': a proclivity to reduce adult organizations to their earliest infantile precursors. Erikson was not alone in his skepticism of psychoanalysis' preoccupation with childhood. Just four years earlier, Hartmann (1955) similarly critiqued the 'genetic fallacy': the false assumption that the continuity of function negates the development of function.

Erikson (1950) accepted Freud's (1905) theory of psychosexual regression. He did not include it, that is, in his critique of originology. At the same time, however, he introduced a potentially subversive theory of modal shifts. The Eriksonian modes—incorporative, retentive-eliminative and intrusive—express familiar unconscious aims (Cf. Freud, 1905). They are not limited, however, to the erotogenic zones. They each reflect a pleasure, beyond that of sexual gratification, in a particular form of mastery or self-assertion. The infant, for example, finds pleasure not just in ingesting breast milk, but in taking in the myriad sounds, smells, sights and sensations of his environment. The toddler likes to use his growing muscles—not just his anal sphincter, but also his legs, arms and hands—to hold on and throw things away. The 5-year-old asserts his prowess by penetrating forbidden spaces—not just, or even primarily, the phantasied mother's body.

The modes are motivational dispositions made possible by bodily maturation and, in that sense, have a phase-specific onset. Once established, they persist and develop in interaction with later modes. The person can shift between them within the same phase of life. Incorporative phantasies might, for example, originate in the oral phase. Oral wishes can then recur, without the implication of regression, in later phases of development. Arlow and Brenner (1964) suggested, to this point, that the oral impulse to eat the analyst might express a genital phase wish to kill and absorb the strength of the father.

The theory of modes indicates that oral or anal phase onset wishes can repeat in later phases, for example, the phallic/genital phases, in qualitatively new (i.e., non-regressive) ways. Moreover, it undermines the reduction of modal behavior to specific erotogenic zones. In this way, it calls into question classical assumptions about what constitutes evidence of a regression. Consider the claim that the incorporation of the lost object in melancholia signals "a regression from object-cathexis to the still narcissistic oral phase of the libido" (Freud, 1917c, p. 250). The oral zone is perhaps the most obvious site of incorporation. But, if we follow Erikson, then the mouth is no more important than, say, the ears, eyes, nose and skin-surface in internalizing the lost object. To expand incorporation beyond the infantile oral zone is to render the proposal of an oral regression unnecessary.

Newer lifespan theories have moved further still from regression logic. They have done so implicitly and without cross-referencing. The trend suggests a growing metapsychological consensus, which, I suggest, cuts across well-established theoretical differences.

Galatzer-Levy and Cohler (1993) argue, for instance, in their self-psychological lifespan theory, that we develop with essential others in each phase toward increased mastery and integrity. Adversity might cause defensive or adaptive 'shifts' in the experience of self and others (p. 341). The term regression itself plays no role in their original contribution. It enters into their account only in their review of previous theories of development (pp. 143, 152, 160, 191). Their limited usage suggests its conceptual irrelevance.

From a Kleinian perspective, Waddell (1998) argues for PS-D shifts across the lifespan. Each major life transition evokes the pain of loss, separation and guilt. At each step, the person retreats (non-regressively) from internal conflict to paranoid-schizoid mechanisms. To develop is, in essence, to mourn loss and endure separateness with courage and integrity. The capacity to face internal conflict with courage depends on the internalization of a containing object whose presence allows for self-soothing and integration.

There are important and well-established differences between ego psychology, self-psychology and Kleinian object relations. Ego psychologists, for instance, tend to value the developmental achievement of autonomy. Self-psychologists, by contrast, prize the developmental achievement of healthy interdependency. Both ego psychologists and self-psychologists reject the death instinct—a universal force in Kleinian thought. Ego psychologists and Kleinians, in turn, reject self psychology's rejection of classical drive theory.

At the same time, each school is capable in principle of accounting for the others' observations. Kohut (1984), for instance, did not deny the existence of the paranoid-schizoid position. He simply re-explained it as a break down product of selfobject rupture. I have written what follows in descriptive language. By this he means we can engage—in common everyday language—with the phenomena that point to irreversible development. It is presupposed that each reader will integrate these findings in his own manner.

Lifespan Issues

Shift logic has gradually displaced regression logic in psychoanalytic lifespan theorizing. A complimentary trend has emerged, meanwhile, in infant research and relational theory: the lifespan issues approach. This approach regards psychopathology as the outcome of cumulative lifespan development. It rejects the traditional approach in which specific pathologies result from phase-specific fixations or deficits. Stern (1985) argued, for example, that we erroneously date core clinical 'issues'—for example, 'autonomy,' 'orality,' 'symbiosis,' 'individuation,' 'trust,' 'attachment,' 'mastery' and 'curiosity'—to problems in early life phases, when, in fact, they play out in each phase of life. Mitchell (1988) held similarly that many 'issues'—for example, 'fusion,' 'separation,' 'dependence' and 'independence'—are not the direct result of any one specific hang-up in childhood, but rather are "basic to the human experience throughout the life cycle" (p. 146). The implication is that one does not regress, but reengages these issues at each phase.

The word *issue* is used here in the common psychological sense: "An emotional or psychological difficulty or problem; a point of emotional conflict" (OED, *Issue*, 16.a). It applies an abstract label to designate a thematic cluster of intrapsychic-interpersonal difficulties. Our lived experience of these difficulties proceeds not through the abstractions themselves, but through the context-specific self-object configurations from which we derive them. The lifespan issues approach contributes not one theory of development, but rather the question, How has this or that issue developed through the lifespan?

Let us consider, for example, the 'merger-hungry' personality (Kohut & Wolf, 1978). The merger-hungry type yearns to break down self–other boundaries. He in fact needs the other—whether a mirror, and ideal or a twin—to fill a deficit in his psychic structure. The other, in his affirming and calming function, is felt to be a needed part of him. To distinguish between self and other is tantamount to losing control over a body part.

"It is only in the light of our appreciation of the crucial influence exerted on the development of the self by the personality of the selfobjects of childhood," the authors write, "that we are able to trace the genetic roots of the disorders of the self" (p. 417). It satisfies a historicizing impulse to date the origins of merger hunger in infantile selfobject ruptures. A lifespan issues approach cannot—and does not want to—debunk this early possibility. It simply asks whether an early deficit is enough to account for the shape and content of the present adult patient's merger fantasies. It suggests that it is *not enough* unless one adds subsequent developmental influences that update and contextualize the yearning.

The lifespan account that follows indicates nodal developmental merger phenomena across the life cycle. The closing vignette provides a concrete illustration of how an adult man's merger hunger evolved from early maternal ruptures through early adult identity seeking.

Timelessness

To re-engage with an old or familiar lifespan issue is not to regress to its first iteration. Through (non-regressive) shifts, the person negotiates evolving issues in each new phase. Still one might picture a hierarchical model (e.g., Gedo, 1979). Infantile motives would play out on the lowest level. New phases would add new levels to the hierarchy. But to preserve this imagery would be to marginalize the critique. It would leave unchallenged the conventional belief that infantile motives underlie all subsequent configurations. The belief itself is embedded in Freud's (1937) archeological vision. It suggests a timeless infantile substratum beneath later geological accretions. Analysis is supposed to lead beneath the superficial residue of the immediate world to these early relics.

A deeper critique of regression necessitates a revised understanding of the timeless unconscious. Freud (1915) described the unconscious as timeless in three senses: Its processes are "not ordered temporally," are "not altered by the passage of time," and "make no reference to time" (p. 186). The first sense—no temporal ordering—is unproblematic. One can develop unconsciously without unconsciously ordering one's life in a temporal narrative. The third sense—no time reference—is not, in fact, a universal property. Some unconscious memories do refer to a specific time. Consider, for instance, the Wolfman's unconscious primal scene memory, which, in Freud's (1909) reconstruction, referred to a scene at 18 months. But nor is it a problem for the critique of regression. Unconscious representations can develop over time whether or not they refer to specific times. Only the second sense—that the unconscious is not altered by the passage of time—presents a problem. It means that we can only conceptualize lifespan development as a layering process: New layers get added onto old ones without changing them.

To discard the concept of regression is implicitly to discard the second sense of timelessness. It is, in essence, to hypothesize that the unconscious develops irreversibly over time. It develops, I suggest, through the constant and pervasive work of deferred action (see Chapter 4). The work of deferred action proceeds, in some cases, through the retranscription, or reconfiguration, of longstanding memories in new context-sensitive forms (Modell, 1990). It works, in other cases, through the first-time transcription of the unformulated (Faimberg, 2007; Stern, 2015). The unconscious does develop over time, if we follow this revision, through the constant transcription and retranscription of internal representations.

The Work of Mourning

The constant work of deferred action implies an ongoing process of loss and mourning in development. Freud (1917c) described mourning as a reaction to the loss of an object, or to the loss of an abstraction, for example, a principle or an ideal, which has replaced an object (p. 243). In the work of mourning, the person must face the loss and detach from the lost object. It is a gradual and prolonged process. "Each single one of the memories and expectations in which the libido is bound to the object," Freud writes, "is brought up and hyper-cathected, and the detachment of the libido is accomplished in respect of it" (p. 245).

The work of mourning is, in Freud's (1917c) formulation, a conscious process. It differs in this regard from melancholia. The melancholic too gives the impression of having lost something or someone, but he typically does not know what it is, or, even if he does recognize "whom he has lost," still does not recognize "what he has lost in him" (p. 244).

The melancholic differs, moreover, from the person in mourning in that the former has become ruthlessly self-critical: "he reproaches himself, vilifies himself and expects to be cast out and punished" (Freud, 1917c, p. 245). To explain the melancholic's self-abasement, Freud proposed that he has withdrawn his libido from the lost object into the ego. The person then identified himself with the lost object. The lost object, Freud elaborated, was a loved and hated figure. When the melancholic identified with this lost object, he turned the hostility and unvoiced criticisms he had once felt toward her upon himself.

Later Freud (1923) turned the process of identification in melancholia into a general principle of development. "When it happens," he wrote, "that a person has to give up a sexual object, there quite often ensues an alteration of his ego which can only be described as a setting up of the object inside the ego, as it occurs in melancholia" (p. 28). He came to regard the process a frequent one, especially in the early phases of development. The character of the ego is, then, a 'precipitate' of lost objects and reflects their history.

The theory of deferred action deepens our sense of the mourning inherent in development. Even the memories by which we preserve our lost objects are themselves lost to time. They are sketched in fading ink and must constantly be redrawn in new ways. There is, therefore, an implicit work of mourning in the act of remembering the past.

The process of mourning in deferred action is more fundamental than the process Freud described. As mentioned, he considered mourning a conscious process. The work of mourning in deferred action is, by contrast, an implicit process in all memory recall. It reflects the inevitable loss that occurs in conscious and unconscious memory formation. It might, but need not, turn into a melancholic state. Often, I suspect the loss inherent in remembering registers not at all, or, perhaps, in a mild sense of lost and irretrievable time.

The resistance to mourning can be so intense, Freud (1917c) wrote, that the person retreats from reality and falls back on wishful thinking to keep the lost object alive in his fantasy. The theory of regression might operate, in this spirit, as an intellectual defense against the irreversible loss of the past implicit in human development. It enables the fantasy of a literal return to past structures of subjectivity, which, in fact, are irretrievably lost.

In Chapter 2, I addressed the morality of maturity by which the analyst locates the most volatile and threatening aspects of human life in co-constructed child in the patient's mind. Now I suggest that, behind any defensive move to disavow the 'childish' elements in one's personality, there lies a deeper wish to return to the time in which they originated. The wish itself might serve defensive or restorative aims. It is keeping alive the fantasy of a return to a lost time it functions, in essence, as a denial of the loss implicit in development.

Novelty and Repetition

Each phase of the lifespan develops the potential latent in earlier phases to produce a qualitatively new—even if in some respects familiar—psychological organization. Nonlinear dynamic systems theorists might describe the new organization as an 'emergent' phenomenon: Old and new phase-specific variables have, in essence, coalesced to generate a qualitatively new system (Galatzer-Levy, 2002). It has never before existed in just this way. Nor was it represented in or pre-determined by a prior stage.

To emphasize novelty is not, as it might seem, to downplay the pervasiveness of repetition. The challenge, for a regression critique, is to theorize familiar, or repetitive, events in a new mental organization, which, by virtue of its newness, is not a return to anything. The study of nonlinear dynamic systems, which originated in math and the hard sciences, has yielded some ways for psychoanalysis to think about repetition in novel contexts (Galatzer-Levy, 1995, 2002, 2004, 2009; Stolorow & Atwood, 1997; Mayes, 2001; Thelen, 2005; Lament, 2013). Its most essential contribution, for my purposes, is to have framed psychopathology neither in terms of infantile fixation, nor of arrest, but in terms of rigidity. The term *rigidity* extends the casual account from infancy to present rigid patterns.

Consider, for example, the case of a young man who suffered from obsessional symptoms—ruminating, counting, obsessive dieting etc.—with flare-ups at nearly every major life transition (his mother's divorce and remarriage in latency, puberty, leaving for college). Mr. A. tended, in session, to retreat from emotional outbursts into intellectual discussion:

> Mr. A. began most analytic sessions with some topic in mind about which he felt strongly. He developed it at some length. (For example,

> he would speak with rage about his father's departure.) After the topic had been engaged, the analyst often made a defense interpretation. (The analyst agreed that the patient was angry with his father for leaving but wondered whether his more immediate anger wasn't addressed to the analyst, who had recently returned from vacation.) At first the patient engaged the interpretation vigorously. ("You always think it's you. You! But you don't think it's you enough not to go on your stupid vacations!") Then the patient began a much less affective, more intellectual discussion of why he had used the identified defense. ("I wonder why I use displacement so much. That is the right term, isn't it?")
> (Galatzer-Levy, 1995, p. 1107)

A regression theorist might search, in this material, for a latent anal fixation (Freud, 1908, 1909, 1913a; Abraham, 1923). Perhaps Mr. A. retreated from a conflict with the Oedipal father-analyst into the obsessional management of emotions that, for him, symbolized feces. A nonlinear approach would not negate the possibility of anal symbolism. It would, however, suggest a nonlinear casual account. It would lead us to search for a rigid 'rule'—one that might generate a complex session without specifying the details in advance (Galatzer-Levy, 2004). One rule might be that *anxiety prompts a retreat into intellectual mastery*. Such a principle might have originated in the mastery of the anal sphincter. It might also have originated in other sites of mastery, for example, waking, grasping and speaking. Nonlinear dynamics does not posit a specific genetic interpretation. It suggests more simply that a procedural rule, such as the above, can evolve beyond its origins. It can generate complexity not contained in or specified by the original conflict site.

Each phase of the life cycle constitutes an emergent landscape of tasks and potentials. Implicit rules, or organizing principles (Stolorow & Atwood, 1984), play out on new developmental landscapes to yield repetitions with new twists. Regression theories tend to label these idiosyncratic repetitions as regression. I want to show, by contrast, that each so-called regression is, in fact, an emergent phenomena in the present field. In each one, we find form and content that emerged only now in the current iteration.

The Phases of the Life Cycle

Each phase of the life cycle closes old doors and opens new developmental potentials. Old patterns reiterate in each new field of possibility. Such re-iteration is often mislabeled 'regression.' In this section I look at how we might reconsider some well-known 'regressions,' *not* as regressions, but as qualitatively novel events of the lifespan.

The infant, to begin, is born with the capacity to start organizing the world of self and others in terms of his invariant behavioral, perceptual and affective experiences (Stern, 1985). The earliest task of development might be simply to organize the world into initial invariant patterns as a precondition for more organized defensive and adaptive activity.

The infant's emergent capacities support a nascent sense of self in relation to others (Stern, 1985). From day one, he begins to develop a physical sense of himself as coherent agent in space and time (Stern, 1985). Over the first two years, he learns to negotiate his and his parents' affects and intentions (Stern, 1985; Galatzer-Levy & Cohler, 1993; BCPSG, 2007). In the back-and-forth, he and the parent shape and re-shape each other's subjective world. Traditionally the infant is thought to fuse, or merge, with the parent. The supposedly merged infant recognizes, according to Stern (1985), that he and his parents are distinct physical agents. Any such merger must then, reflect an affective mix-up: a feeling that, although physically separate, we feel and want the same things.

Patients often express a dread of losing themselves in the analyst's experiential world. Many fear regressing, some analysts would hold, to a vulnerable site of mother–infant trauma: a hard object in the mother–infant mix-up (Balint, 1968), an impingement in the holding environment (Winnicott, 1965), or archaic selfobject rupture (Kohut, 1971). The patient does not, however, return to the infant–parent mix-up in its original form. The wish to merge—and the dread—reflect a lifelong history of joyful and traumatic mix-ups. In what follows, I point out later mergers in adolescent hero worship, in mutual intimacy and in becoming a parent. (A detailed account would mention others still.) I then show, for illustration, how one man's adolescent wish to become an artist re-conditioned whatever might have been his original yearning to be at one with his illusive mother.

Through inevitable ruptures and separations, the child learns, in optimal development, to tolerate frustration, delay, transience and loss. Here the Kleinian tradition emphasizes the relevant crucible of weaning. "Weaning can be thought of as the prototype," Waddell (1998) writes,

> for all separations and losses. . . . It stirs anew every early experience of being cut off from what is felt to be the primary source of love and

> sustenance; of being left alone when company was needed; of being starved when food was required; of being deprived of a cohering presence when holding was wanted.
>
> (p. 62)

The adult who rages at normal delays and frustrations does often seem like a baby. The loss of the breast is, however, in the present theory, the loss of an ever-evolving psychic object. To lose a lover was, in the following case of Travis, not simply to lose his mother's breast, but to lose a muse—a condensation of maternal and later self-images.

In moving from infancy to toddlerhood, the child develops muscular control and coordination. He can grasp objects and let them go (Erikson, 1950), control his anal sphincter (Freud, 1905; Abraham, 1923; Shengold, 1985), crawl and walk further and further (Mahler, 1975). Bodily maturation promotes a feeling of autonomy, mastery and independence. The parent expects him to use his new agency to obey rules. It becomes meaningful to defy or comply with expectations. With greater autonomy also comes separation anxiety and guilt (Mahler, 1975). Perceived failure can result in shame and doubt (Erikson, 1950). Stubborn, willful, defiant and obsessive adults are reminiscent of a toilet training toddler. Classical theory took such behavior as evidence of an anal regression (Freud, 1908; Abraham, 1923; Shengold, 1985). In this regard, it privileges anality. The anal sphincter is, however, but one site of an overall increase in physical mastery. The gain in overall mastery—not just in anal control—make possible the behavior in question. What it means to control this or that evolves over time. Even shit, to use the classical example, develops as a psychic object with ever-new meanings and associations. Feldman (1999), to this point, presents a patient for whom messiness means a muddled mind. The patient associates it with two disorganized colleagues and suddenly his analyst. It is unlikely for a toddler to make such abstract metaphorical links (Rizzolo, 2017).

In the midst of the mastery drama, toddlers often face in reality—and perhaps always in phantasy (Mitchell, 2013)—a sibling birth. He learns, in what Mitchell terms sibling trauma, that he is no longer the baby. Some toddlers repress jealousy and hatred for the new arrival beneath an overt wish for closeness. Others fight to get back their old status. Some give up speech, eating habits, toilet training and walking in a 'regression' to babyhood (Mitchell, 2013). The toddler becomes at once "baby and big girl/big boy" (p. 29). One might question, however, what the regression is a return to. The baby/big-girl split did not exist in infancy. It is an emergent structure. One might isolate the 'baby' part as the 'regressed' part of the mind. But in so far as it exists in an internal dialectic with 'big girl,' the new 'baby' self is not a pure replica of the actual past baby self.[3]

Around age three, the child, in the classical account, enters the Oedipal situation (Freud, 1924). Klein (1928, 1945) located it in the first year. Timing aside, it means the entry into a love triangle. The Oedipal child asserts himself as each parent's rival for the other. The healthy parent can enjoy his gestures and attacks without too much seduction or retaliation (Kohut, 1977; Terman, 1984). The Oedipal patient might imagine himself in a rivalry with the analyst for the love and adoration of the world's women. The female patient might imagine that she interests or enlivens the analyst in a way that his wife does not. The Oedipal adult patient has not regressed, however, to the original situation. It is a new version.[4] At the very least, the conditions have changed. For the child to win the Oedipal contest is, for instance, a trauma. The father is dethroned. The mother is shown to be needy and seductive. The child learns to dread the external efficacy of his private phantasies. For the adult, by contrast, victory is *not* a trauma. It is possible and indeed likely that he will, for instance, become more appealing than his father/analyst to his future wife. In phantasy, he then gets a mother to himself (Klein, 1959). The satisfaction softens his competitiveness and allows for a more benign relationship with his internal father.

In latency, the world expands beyond the family of origin to include the broader community. The child becomes more invested in peer acceptance and extra-familial authority figures (Galatzer-Levy & Cohler, 1993). He also makes gains in conceptual abstraction (Harter, 1986). The child therefore internalizes the expanded object world into an increasingly sophisticated phantasy life. He relies on phantasy to express his impulses before growth in puberty opens up greater potential to enact them (Sarnoff, 1976). He does, however, express a nascent action potential in his entry into the 'tool world' (Erikson, 1950). In play, he engages the skills and technologies valued in his culture.

Bornstein (1951) observed a passive, clingy, obsessive disposition in latency children. She proposed that they had regressed from sexual and aggressive conflict to pre-genitality. But nothing justifies the assumption that such overt behavior is inherently pre-genital. Psychoanalysis seeks to understand its meaning—and meaning develops across the lifespan (Rizzolo, 2016). In early childhood, it is acceptable and often cute, for instance, to be passive and clingy. It is a good way of getting love. In latency, the same behavior becomes shameful. The child becomes a 'mamma's boy.' He faces not only his peers' ridicule, but also his parent's concern and often their unconscious disappointment. He internalizes the response in a newly emergent structure of self-contempt.

Physical and social changes in puberty open new potentials for sexual and aggressive enactment (Waddell, 1998). To manage his impulses, and so avert real danger, the adolescent turns, Anna Freud (1936) observed, to intellectualization and (inconsistent) asceticism. He tries to work out his phantasies in fields of cognitive abstraction. He tries, on more personal terms, to renounce his wishes and so establish his moral superiority. Of course, he fails. He falls often into turbulent enactments in which he tries to work out his internal problems by moving around the external figures who embody them (Galatzer-Levy & Cohler, 1993). It becomes all the more urgent, to the extent that he sees himself in his objects, to renounce his desires and regain his superior position.

The adolescent routinely orchestrates new situations reminiscent of earlier traumas. Some theorists regard the re-enactments as regressions. "Regression in adolescence," Bloss (1967) writes, "is the precondition for progressive development" (p. 177). By re-creating 'miniature editions' of old situations he brings "more extended resources" to master "prototypical danger situations." The re-enactment is not, however, a return to the original situation. The adolescent brings *new resources* to bear on the situation. He can, for instance, use his intellect to anticipate and contain once overwhelming affect. The implicit reflective function renders the new experience more manageable. We find one example, albeit in an older patient, in the case of Travis. (To develop through miniature re-enactments is certainly not the sole prerogative of the adolescent.)

With further education, and in the face of increased social expectation, the emerging adult enters the world of work. He might worry consciously about what or who he should become, manifest, most obviously, in a vocational direction. Beneath his conscious worry, he must unconsciously integrate his potentials and identifications into a work-identity. I use the term *work-identity* instead of 'ego-identity' (Erikson, 1950), because I want to specify the way in which this phase contributes to lifelong identity formation. To establish a work-identity is, on an unconscious level, to emphasize certain potentials over others (Levenson, 1978). Once prized pursuits will—with much pain, doubt and self-recrimination—become hobbies or after-hours side-projects. It is painful to abandon them, or to marginalize them, not just because of their intrinsic value, but because they express needed internal object-ties. To abandon a once prized path is to abandon the internal object-ties—and idealized self-representations—expressed in the pursuit.

To choose a path is, then, to mourn others not taken. It is, moreover, to endure a narcissistic injury: The person must accept the limitations inherent in self-definition. He cannot actualize his every potential. If he wants to succeed, he must focus his energy and attention. A former sense of unlimited potential must be channeled into practical goals and ambitions. Some resist the pressure to choose something. The person who refuses to make a choice, preferring to "keep his options open," often finds himself stagnant, watching his peers progress in their careers, unable to commit to any of his various dreams.

The young adult might retreat from identity crisis into an intense dependency on the analyst. He looks to the analyst to understand and guide him much like the parent of infancy. "In this they truly regress," Erikson wrote,

> for either openly or covertly they expect from the therapist the kind of omniscience an infant attributes to his mother when he seems to assume that she should have prevented the table from hitting him, or at any rate from being hard and sharp; or that she should be able to hold him firmly and to let him go freely at the same time, that is, at a time when he himself does not know which he wants.
>
> (p. 103)

The merger functions, however, in the unique context of the adult present. It is here, for instance, that the patient might discover her own wish to become therapist. Some find themselves listening and interpreting to the friends in the therapist's style. Others fantasize in less obvious ways about incorporating the therapist's analytic identity, for example, her calm, her steadiness, her understanding, her investment in meaningful work etc. The patient imagines that she can pass through the therapist—a kind of transformational object (Bollas, 1979)—into a clarified sense of potential, direction and agency.

Beyond a work-identity, the young adult—out of loneliness, social pressure, a new sense of maturity, and a vaguely formulated readiness for a commitment—must develop a capacity for romantic intimacy (Erikson, 1950, 1968) or marriage (Waddell, 1998). Unlike most past intimacies—e.g., child/parent, child/teacher—romantic intimacy is symmetrical. The partners bear an equal devotion to and responsibility for each other's wellbeing. They must be able to suppress actions and forgo pleasures that would betray the relationship. They must learn, moreover, to surrender to an emergent intersubjective rhythm (Ghent, 1990). The readiness for such reciprocity depends on a solidity in ones' identity (Erikson, 1950). Without a firm, if fluid, sense of self, the pursuit of intimacy becomes, in essence, a search for identity. The fear of submission, of getting lost in the wrong identity, of turning into an extension of the other etc., leads to conflict and ruptures.

The reciprocal lover-to-lover rhythm has a certain similarity to the mother–infant rhythm. Some regression theorists emphasize the similarity. Ferenczi (1938), for instance, interpreted sexual intimacy as the expression of a regressive wish to return to the womb. The penis, by his account, symbolizes the male self. The vagina symbolizes the womb. By implication the woman, who becomes the mother, is denied her own yearning for maternal containment. (In compensation, she gets a baby.) Lovers do play parent to each other. The parent–child bond was, however, an asymmetrical bond of power and responsibility. The lover's play occurs, by contrast, in a symmetrical context. The woman might contain the 'child in the man.' The man might hold and cherish the 'child in the woman.' In a healthy couple, the roles shift back and forth. In nurturing and being nurtured, the lovers, as Klein (1959) observed, enable a reworking of internal objects. To get the new phantasied mother to oneself can, for instance, temper the jealousy the man perhaps felt in childhood toward his father or siblings—potential rivals for the actual childhood mother's attention—and, in effect, recast the internal mother as more available. To play the father to his wife, meanwhile, can bolster the young husband's confidence in his masculinity and give rise to a more equal relation to one's internal father. The symmetry of care—playing both child and parent—renders it a new experience.

In becoming a parent, the person enters an even more complex developmental landscape. Parenthood is a developmental phase, in Benedek's (1959) classic account, *because* of its regressive potential. The parent, she held, regresses to the child's phase of development. The breast-feeding mother regresses, for instance, to her own oral needs and fixations. The regression helps her, in the best of cases, to identify with and intuit her child's needs. It enables her, moreover, to rework her own early traumas from a new vantage point of agency, understanding and mastery. The internal split (self-as-actual-mother/self-as-phantasied-child) is, however, new to the parent's psychology. It is not a return to anything. The phantasied child-self, for one, does not reflect a direct reliving of her early life. It represents an idiosyncratic remembrance in light of the current child. It is, moreover, a reversal of the original parent–child asymmetry. She now holds the power and responsibility. She can better parent her child, and in a sense, better parent herself in the identification. In parenting herself, she can repair internal child representations and, at the same time, soften her own parental introjects—which now expand to include her example.

In emphasizing the child's dependency on significant adults, psychoanalysis tends to minimize the adult's reciprocal dependence on children and younger adults (Erikson, 1950). The healthy midlife adult develops a 'generative' interest in guiding the next generation. He does not out of pure altruism, but out of the narcissistic wish to leave a legacy. Implicitly, he recognizes his aging and eventual death. He depends on younger generations to affirm him. It is uncomfortable to need the young people he wants to be needed by. Some evade the discomfort through a self-derision by which they disavow the wish to be needed. Others reject their mentees' idealization for fear of indulging it too much (Galatzer-Levy & Cohler, 1993). Others still exploit their mentee's adoration, inciting and cultivating it, feeling vaguely betrayed when the younger person outgrows them.

When generative strivings fail, Erikson (1950) wrote, we sometimes observe a "regression to an obsessive need for pseudo-intimacy," marked by "a pervading sense of stagnation and personal impoverishment" (p. 267). The partners in a pseudo-intimacy indulge themselves, "as if there were their own—or one another's—one and only child." One might question, though, what this 'regression' is a regression to. The younger adult developed, in the ideal scenario, a capacity for genuine intimacy—the ability to establish and maintain a symmetrical love relationship. It was not an evasion, but an entry into life. The midlife adult, by contrast, *retreats* from feelings of insignificance into defensive indulgence. It is a two-way enactment by which he and his partner avoid narcissistic vulnerability.

In the last years of life, the person normatively faces retirement, physical and sometimes mental decline, and the more frequent death of loved ones. He must draw, more overtly than in past phases, on the capacity to tolerate loss and transience (Waddell, 1998). The capacity to tolerate loss depends, in part, on the ability to narrate one's life coherently (Galatzer-Levy & Cohler, 1993). In the telling, and re-telling, the person struggles to accept his "one and only life," including the frustrations, with a sense of integrity and resolution (Erikson, 1950, p. 268). It is the final act of mourning, integration, gratitude and forgiveness for one's own and other's faults—often carried out over years—before death.

End-of-life adults often regress, some hold, to infantile neediness, obsessional latency-age behavior, or moody adolescent defiance (Waddell, 1998). Old people do sometimes behave in a childlike way. The question is whether they regress. The aging adult often finds himself, like the infant, intensely dependent on others for basic physical care. Unlike the infant, however, the adult has experienced physical autonomy. The *loss* of autonomy, implicit in the aging adult's neediness, opens a new end-of-life mourning process.

Obsessional and defiant behavior also take on new meaning in the face of death's approach. The latency child might have become obsessional in his zeal to master the tool world. The adolescent might have become defiant out of a wish to establish his independence. Their outlook was future oriented. The elder adult, by contrast, must accept his past. Those who lived poorly, or who never lived, often feel despair, manifest as disgust (Erikson, 1950). "Time is now short," Erikson writes, "too short for the attempt to start another life and to try out alternate roads to integrity. Disgust hides despair, if only in the form of 'a thousand little disgusts'" (p. 269). The adult might retreat into obsessional or defiant behavior. The retreat, however, is not exactly a return. It is imbued with a past-oriented feeling-tone—disgust, despair, regret—that renders it a new experience. The work—to accept one's life-as-lived—is, at this point, an unprecedented task.

Conclusion

The person progresses irreversibly through the lifespan. He shifts back and forth, for self-protective and adaptive purposes, between alternate configurations of desire and defense. Through shifting configurations, he engages with persistent lifespan problems. Historically psychoanalysis emphasized the likeness between childhood and adult problems. The present account suggests that they also differ in meaningful ways. The person brings his childhood internalizations forwards, through deferred action, in a new way that reflects the wishes, needs, tasks and pressures of the present. In each new phase, we find the repetition of the familiar in a novel emergent configuration. There is no going back. In this sense, the work of development is, as Freud (1923) held, a work of mourning.

Notes

1 An earlier version of this chapter has been accepted for publication in *The Psychoanalytic Study of the Child* (Rizzolo, in press).
2 An earlier version of this chapter featuring material from both Chapters 5 and 10 has been accepted for publication in *The Psychoanalytic Study of the Child* (Rizzolo, 2018, in press at time of writing). It is reprinted here and expanded into two separate chapters by permission of the journal and Yale University Press.
3 The critique of regression relies on the basic proposition that one cannot understand a "part" of the mind in isolation from mind-as-a-whole (Rizzolo, 2016). If we could, then we could always isolate just that part reminiscent of the old self. We could call it the regressed part. But we would have ruled out a-priori any new variables.
4 Britton (1992) similarly writes that the Oedipal is never resolved but must be re-worked at each new stage of development.

Chapter 6

The Specter of the Primitive[1]

Traditional psychoanalytic theories of development hold that the adult neurotic can regress, or has already regressed, to the childhood arrests and/or fixations in which his pathology originated. More recent critiques have called this possibility into question (Stolorow, Brandchaft, & Atwood, 1987; Mitchell, 1988; Inderbitzin & Levy, 2000; Rizzolo, 2016). It is unlikely that anyone can roll back the additions and modifications of lifespan development in a full-fledged return to the needs, wishes and anxieties of his childhood.

By *regression*, though, some analysts mean not a full-fledged return to an earlier developmental phase, but a non-phase-specific slip into primitive fantasies and defenses. The operational term, in this particular variation, is not *regression* but *primitive*. It appears most often in Kleinian and Kleinian-inspired traditions. The shift from the depressive to the paranoid-schizoid position is, for instance, considered not a phase-specific regression, but a regression to primitive forms of mentation (Klein, 1946, p. 15).

The concept of primitivity in psychoanalysis originated in Freud's equation (1900, 1912–1913) of the neurotic with the aboriginal subject portrayed in late nineteenth to early twentieth century anthropology (Tylor, 1871; Smith, 1894; Frazer, 1910, 1911–1915). Of particular consequence was the link Freud (1912–1913) drew from primitive magic in Tylor to the "omnipotence of thoughts"—which was the Rat Man's term—in modern neurotic disorders (p. 84). The intermediary link was the child. If one takes literally the claim that ontogeny recapitulates phylogeny, then the regressed analysand becomes a psychological child who preserves, in turn, the thought patterns of our prehistoric ancestors.

Freud's phylogenetic story, and the underlying principle of recapitulation, have long been disproven (Boas, 1928; Gertz, 1973; Cole & Scribner, 1974; Gould, 1977). We nonetheless find their traces preserved in contemporary psychoanalytic approaches to what are termed the 'primary' processes and 'primitive' defenses. Hinshelwood (1991) writes, for example, that, "one of the most important characteristics of the primitive defense mechanisms is the quality of *omnipotence*, which gives rise to major changes in the structure of the mind and personality" (p. 124; emphasis added). The magical quality and animistic undertones of the so-called primitive defenses (as seen, for instance, in projective identification) preserve a metaphorical connection with Freud's vision of the aboriginal subject.

In this chapter, I argue that the 'primary' processes and 'primitive' defenses are not primitive. That is, they are neither evolutionarily nor developmentally primary. I will first address the erroneous claim that primary process and primitive forms of mentation—as observed in the modern analyst's consulting room—are representative of the mental processes of prehistoric humans. The claim itself stems from a Darwinian effort in the nineteenth-century social sciences—now discredited—to order cultures and their people in a hierarchy of social adaptation according to the principle of survival of the fittest (Cole & Scribner, 1974). The mistake in such an approach, which Boas (1928) and Gertz (1973) have articulated, was to treat the scientific progress of America and Western Europe as evidence for the superior mental capacities of American and Western European adults. It was *as if* the Western adult subject had achieved greater individual capacity for adaptive 'secondary' process thought. By reverse logic, the less adaptive mental processes of the child and the mental patient were considered templates for the primitive thought patterns of our ancestors.

Today most analysts would presumably reject any echoes of social Darwinism. Yet many would still argue that primary processes and primitive defenses are, if not uniquely characteristic of prehistoric man, still characteristic of infantile mentation. To do so is to jettison Freud's phylogenetic claim but retain the developmental claim.

Later in what follows, I will deconstruct this effort to salvage the term *primitive*. Are the primary processes and primitive defenses indeed elemental, or primary, in infantile development? I argue, again in the negative, that they are not. I first demonstrate that, even by Freud's own lights, hallucinatory wish fulfillment—the defining operation of the primitive mind—is not a primary infantile operation. Any infantile hallucination presupposes a nonhallucinatory experience of reality (Freud, 1900; Hartmann, 1939; Fairbairn, 1952; Stern, 1985; Lear, 1998; Erreich, 2003). This means that hallucinatory wish fulfillment is a secondary, or derivative, phenomenon. I argue, second, that splitting and projective identification—the core primitive defenses in Kleinian theory—are not inherently infantile, but rather develop across the life cycle. They do so as a function of development in the capacity for abstract thinking, which in turn allows for greater play in what the person yokes together and how he splits or projects it. The result is lifespan development in the so-called primitive defenses.

Psychoanalysis should, by implication, discard the concept of primitivity. Any fantasy of an analyst's cultural superiority over the primitive patient must be explored, if it emerges, for context-specific countertransference meanings. We require, beyond this point, a lifespan approach to hallucinatory wish fulfillment, splitting and projective identification. To engage in them is not to indulge in infantile thought patterns, but to make use of increasingly sophisticated mental operations in response to changing real-life contexts.

The Primitive Neurotic

Freud (1900) asserted, in his early discussion of regression, that "what is older in time is more primitive in form" (p. 548). By primitive, he meant early both in the lifespan and in human history. He relied here on the Haeckelian principle[2] that ontogeny recapitulates phylogeny (Gould, 1977). 'Each individual,' Freud (1916–1917) later wrote, "somehow recapitulates in an abbreviated form the entire development of the human race" (p. 199). The child and the regressed neurotic thus retain the anlagen of primitive times.

The stage was set, then, for a comparison between neurotic mentation and primitive culture. Freud articulated the link in *Totem and Taboo* (1912–1913), subtitled *Some Points of Agreement between the Mental Lives of Savages and Neurotics*. The modern-day 'savage' was taken to represent the early condition of mankind. "There are men still living," in Freud's words (1913b), "who . . . stand very near to primitive man, far nearer than we do, and whom we therefore regard as his direct heirs and representatives. Such is our view of those whom we describe as savages" (p. 1). Freud pointed, first and foremost, to the aboriginal people of Australia.[3] They did not build houses; they did not farm; they did not raise livestock; they were unacquainted with the art of pottery; they worshiped totem animals; and they were terrified of incest. They were devoid, in other words, of the scientific, technological, social and moral refinements of modern Western European and American culture. They were, in Freud's thinking, the "most backward and miserable of savages," children of the "youngest continent, in whose fauna, too we can still observe much that is archaic."

Freud (1912–1913) grounded his phylogenetic theory in early twentieth-century anthropology, especially the work of Tylor (1871), Smith (1894) and Frazer (1910, 1911–1915). He posited a continuity from the animistic religion in Tylor's account of primitive peoples to what he considered the modern-day infant's belief in omnipotent thoughts. Animism, according to Tylor (1871), was the earliest belief system of primitive peoples. It held that "spiritual beings . . . affect or control the events of the material world" (p. 385). Magical thinking played a central role. Primitive man believed he could use 'magic arts' to appeal to the spirit world and so make things happen in the real world (p. 105). Freud (1912–1913) noted this point. "We are not surprised to learn," he wrote, "that, hand in hand with the animistic system, there went a body of instructions upon how to obtain mastery over men, beasts and things—or rather over their spirits" (p. 77). For support he cited Frazer's many examples: nightly rituals to ensure the safe passage of the Egyptian sun-god Ra, rain rituals in Japan, fertility rituals in Java, hunting rituals in Dyak villages (1911–1915). He then leapt from primitive man to childhood development. 'Children,' he held, "are in an analogous psychical situation. . . . they satisfy their wishes in a hallucinatory manner" (p. 84). The prime example was the hallucinatory breast (Freud, 1900, 1911). The modern child preserves the primitive adult's mindset in his belief that—through hallucination or magical thinking—he can make his wishes come true.

From the child Freud turned to the contemporary adult neurotic. He proposed that neurotics—like primitive man and like modern children—indulge in what he now termed the "omnipotence of thoughts" (Freud, 1912–1913, p. 84). He borrowed this term from the Rat Man:

> He had coined the phrase as an explanation of all the strange and uncanny events by which he, like others afflicted with the same illness,

> seemed to be pursued. If he thought of someone, he would be sure to meet that very person immediately afterwards, as though by magic. If he suddenly asked after the health of an acquaintance whom he had not seen for a long time, he would hear that he had just died, so that it would look as though a telepathic message had arrived from him. If, without really serious intention, he swore at some stranger, he might be sure that the man would die soon afterwards, so that he would feel responsible for his death.
>
> (p. 85)

By his fears, the obsessional thus "reveals his resemblance to the savages who believe they can alter the external world by mere thinking" (p. 87). A line was thus drawn from primitive magic to childhood hallucination to omnipotent thinking in the regressed adult neurotic.

Having established this line, Freud sought to account for what he considered mankind's evolution from primitive times to the achievements of modern Western science. Here he joined a long tradition of nineteenth-century European intellectuals who had sought to establish a line of cultural evolution from primitive man to American and European culture (Comte, 1830; Tylor, 1871; Spencer, 1898). Tylor, Freud's most immediate anthropological reference, argued for a cultural progression from the primitive reliance on magical spells to crude tools to the advanced sciences and industrial production capacity in the putatively more mature societies of America and Western Europe. From their reliance on 'sharp stones' and the 'rudest natural bludgeons' humans progressed, Tylor wrote, to carving and shaping wood tools and from there on to metallurgy (p. 59). The assumption was that scientific advances indicate cultural maturation.

Freud went deeper than Tylor in articulating a narrative of psychological progress to explain the supposed cultural progress from primitive times to Western European culture. This psychological progress lay, according to Freud (1912–1913), in the progression from primitive man's magical thinking to modern man's capacity for rational, adaptive thought. In the most primitive phase of cultural evolution, the 'animistic' stage, which Freud believed ran parallel to infantile narcissism, men "ascribed omnipotence to themselves" (p. 87). In a subsequent 'religious' stage, which he linked to the child's idealization of the parents, men transferred their original feeling of omnipotence to the gods. In the final, 'scientific' phase, which Freud considered the most mature, man "renounced the pleasure principle, adjusted himself to reality, and turned to the external world for the object of his desires" (p. 89). The scientific achievements of the West were thought to depend, therefore, on mankind's progression from magical thinking to reality-testing.

The development of reality-testing intersected, in Freud's narrative, with the development of morality. A primitive father, he argued, had once oppressed his sons and kept the tribe's women for himself (Freud, 1912–1913). One day, his sons joined together and killed him. Afterwards they devoured him in order to absorb his strength. Their later remorse and rivalry over the women led to a collective prohibition against murder and incest—the first legal system. To substantiate his claim, Freud pointed to William Robertson Smith's account (1894) of the sacrifice and consumption of totem animals in primitive cultures. 'The totem animal,' Freud wrote, "is in reality a substitute for the father, and this tallies with the contradictory fact that, though the killing of the animal is as a rule forbidden, yet its killing is a festive occasion—with the fact that it is killed and yet mourned" (p. 140).

Today the Freudian child recapitulates the Oedipus drama en route to superego formation (Freud, 1924). The little boy, according to the theory, avoids castration anxiety by relinquishing his sexual interest in his mother and identifying with his father's moral authority. The internal prohibition against patricide and incest recapitulates the original prohibition, established by the primal horde, against their earlier deeds. The ego-ideal thus links him through 'phylogenetic acquisition' to his 'archaic heritage' (Freud, 1923, p. 36).

By implication the pre-Oedipal child is analogous to the violent savage of the primal horde—the primitive subject before the achievement of personal or social morality. Melanie Klein (1946) developed this implication, as I will argue, into a theory of 'primitive' pre-Oedipal defenses characterized, at least in part, by their violent nature.

Tylor (1871) had held that, even in the midst of modern Europe, one could find 'survivors,' individuals who preserved in their way of life the essential nature of more primitive times. The Freudian neurotic became something like the Tylorian survivor. Indeed, Freud took the notion of the survivor more literally than is generally recognized. In 1983, Ilse Grubrich-Simitis discovered an unknown draft of Freud's twelfth metapsychological paper, up to then unpublished, in a trunk given by Ferenczi to Michael Balint. The paper attempts to order different neurotics along the timeline of human evolution. Anxiety hysteria is framed as a residue of primitive man's anxiety in the Ice Age, when the 'friendly' world morphed into "a mass of threatening perils" (Freud, 1915a, p. 14). Conversion hysteria is derived from primitive man's prohibition against genital sex to limit the number of hungry mouths to feed (p. 15). Obsessional neurosis recapitulates a later time when primitive man learned to manipulate the world by thoughts (p. 16). Dementia praecox, which involves a retreat from object-libido, recapitulates the second generation son's experience of being castrated by the primal father (p. 17). Some of the sons escaped castration and fled to form their own community. They subsequently became their own lovers. The paranoiac, who projects his homoerotic wish to be penetrated and then fears it as a threat, recapitulates their homoerotism (p. 18). Melancholia-mania, finally, repeats the depression-elation after the sons killed the primal father. That Freud did not publish the draft perhaps indicates his own doubts. It nonetheless indicates the logical extreme of a view in which two things happen: (1) The history of the individual repeats that of the human race; (2) fixations along the line of phylogenetic/ontogenetic development manifest in modern-day neurotic conditions.

From Speculative Anthropology to Current Metapsychology

Many psychoanalysts would consider Freud's phylogenetic hypotheses speculative and ultimately perhaps irrelevant to the clinical application/evaluation of his model of mind. Freud incorporated aspects of his phylogenetic theory, however, into his model of mind in subtle ways that persist without clear recognition of their anthropological origins. Later theorists, particularly Melanie Klein, extended Freud's theory of primitive man to the study of early defenses. I will focus, for their central role, on the legacy of primitive man in Freud's primary processes (1915a) and in Klein's primitive defenses (1946).

The idea of primitivity enters, to begin, into Freud's still prevalent theory of dream work. "We call it 'regression,'" Freud (1900) wrote, "when in a dream an idea is turned back into the sensory image from which it was originally derived" (p. 543). The regression revives a picture-language considered less mature than verbal expression. The revival of this picture-language promises, in turn, a "picture of a phylogenetic childhood, a picture of the human race, of which the individual's development is in fact an abbreviated recapitulation influenced by the chance circumstances of life" (p. 547). By means of the dream work (e.g., condensation and displacement) and the properties of the unconscious (e.g., timelessness and the absence of negation) the dreamer arranges the dream images to obtain an omnipotent hallucinatory gratification.

The same mechanisms and properties appear later in the theory of primary process (Freud, 1915a). The primary process mind works, like the dream work—and allegedly like the primitive adult—to manipulate the world through slippery chains of loosely connected omnipotent thoughts. Freud (1915b) asserts that "the content of the *Ucs* may be compared with an aboriginal population in the mind" (p. 194). It appears, however, that it is not only the *content,* but also the *processes* of unconscious mentation that enable the comparison. In a recapitulation of human evolution, the exigencies of reality ultimately compel the child to abandon hallucinatory gratification and adopt the reality principle (Freud, 1911).

Freud (1926) suggested that "before its sharp cleavage into and ego and an id, and before the formation of a superego, the mental apparatus makes use of different methods of defense from those which it employs after it has reached these stages of organization" (p. 163). Anna Freud offered some clarification in her comment that "the earliest defense mechanisms of the ego are based on primary processes" (Sandler & Freud, 1983, p. 48). Melanie Klein (1930), by contrast, went beyond clarification to articulate an original theory of primitive defenses—most notably, splitting and projective identification.

Klein (1927) asserted, with Freud, that the "individual repeats biologically the development of mankind" manifest in "stages we still observe in primitive people" (p. 170). If we ask what makes her primitive ego mechanisms 'primitive,' though, we run into the problem of language: "The description of such primitive processes suffers from a great handicap, for these fantasies arise at a time when the infant has not yet begun to think in words" (Klein, 1946, p. 8n). The meaning of primitivity, then, must be derived from somewhere other than the patient's verbal content. I argue that Freud's phylogenetic narrative, which Klein accepted, plays a significant, if unrecognized, role in shaping her usage.

To address the question "What makes primitive defenses primitive?" we must first consider the role of aggression, or sadism, in the Kleinian vision of primitive psychology. Hinshelwood (1991) explains that, in Klein's thought, primitive defense mechanisms are mobilized against anxiety in response to impulses derivative of the death instinct. The mechanisms themselves are charged with a sadism equivalent to the masochism they rebuff. "The excess of sadism," in Klein's words (1930), "gives rise to anxiety and sets in motion the ego's earliest modes of defence" (p. 220). The 'violent character' of these defenses therefore distinguishes them from more mature, tempered defenses.

The notion that primitive defenses are primitive, at least in part, because of their aggressive character raises the further question, What is uniquely primitive about being aggressive? Is it fair to say that primitive cultures were more aggressive than modern ones? Arguably, human beings are as aggressive today as they ever were, but they are armed now with more dangerous weapons.

The notion that primitive man was more aggressive than we are today reflects the enduring influence of Freud's phylogenetic narrative. The lingering assumption is that primitive man was a pre-superego creature. Free from the constraints of conscience, he supposedly expressed his sadistic impulses wildly and without discretion. The child supposedly recapitulates the sadism of primitive man before primitive man acquired a superego, the "cultured part of the personality," that would inhibit his aggressive display (Klein, 1930, p. 170). Unchecked sadism thus becomes a defining feature of the primitive mindset. The cultural prejudice of the West is nowhere clearer than in this theoretical move to designate as 'primitive' the hostile forces that disrupt our otherwise mature society. An alternative would be to say that human nature has always included an aggressive potential—manifest in all cultures—and at all phases of the individual lifespan.

In addition, the primitive defenses are considered primitive because of their omnipotent quality: They distort reality in a manner that suggests total control over the environment. This omnipotent quality connects them back to Freud's account of magical thinking, which, as discussed, linked the primitive man to the hallucinating infant. Indeed, Klein (1946) argued that we need her theory of primitive defenses to explain the infant's hallucinatory breast. The infant, she argues, splits the breast into a good breast and a bad breast. In her account, the infant then denies the existence of the bad breast. The denial implies "a strong feeling of omnipotence—an essential characteristic of early mentality" (p. 7). For Klein, then, the primitive defenses are the very gears that facilitate what Freud considered the quintessential primitive mental operation—wishful thinking.

Tylor (1871) and Freud (1912–1913) traced the progression of culture, as we have seen, from the primitive reliance on magic and crude tools to civilized scientific/technological mastery. The advanced production techniques of Western industrialization colored, in retrospect, what became the crude tools and weapons—and the crude underlying mental operations—of early man. In addition to their omnipotent quality, the primitive defenses evidence a certain crudeness that evokes the imagery of the blunt weapons of primitive culture. Indeed Freud (1900) wrote, in one suggestive passage, that the "primitive weapons, the bows and arrows, that have been abandoned by adult men, turn up once more in the nursery" (p. 567). The primitive defenses of splitting and projective identification, in Kleinian theory, threaten with annihilation the very ego they defend (Hinshelwood, 1991). Blunt and unwieldy tools, they inflict indiscriminate damage, unlike the more sophisticated instruments and, by analogy, more mature mental mechanisms of modern man. The primitive defenses are 'primitive,' then, by analogy with the weapons of early humans.

Tylor (1871), lastly, describes the primitive belief that the soul can "enter into, possess, and act in the bodies of other men, of animals, and even of things" (p. 387). The concept of projective identification suggests a belief of this kind in the infant–mother relation:

> The [child's] phantasied onslaughts on the mother follow two main lines: one is the predominantly oral impulse to suck dry, bite up, scoop out and rob the mother's body of its good contents. . . . The other line of attack derives from the anal and urethral impulses and implies expelling dangerous substances (excrements) out of the self and into the mother. Together with these harmful excrements, expelled in hatred, split-off parts of the ego are also projected onto the mother or, as I would rather call it, *into* the mother. These excrements and bad parts of the self are meant not only to injure but also to control and to take possession of the object. In so far as the mother comes to contain the bad parts of the self, she is not felt to be a separate individual but is felt to be *the* bad self.
>
> (Klein, 1946, p. 8)

The infant in Klein's account, like the primitive adult in Tylor's, imagines he can expel parts of the self into the other in order to injure, control and take possession. The mechanism of projective identification thus preserves a substrate of primitive animism.

We find resonances of Freud's and Klein's accounts in pockets of mid-twentieth-century ego psychology. "Regarding the earliest types of identifications," Jacobson (1964) writes, "magic as they are by nature, they are founded on primitive mechanisms of introjection and projection corresponding to fusions of self and object images which disregard the realistic differences between the self and the object" (pp. 45–46). 'Primitive denial,' Kernberg (1976) writes, from a complementary perspective, "refers to the tendency to see external objects as totally good, in order to make sure that they can protect one against the 'bad' objects, that they cannot be contaminated, spoiled, or destroyed by one's own aggression" (p. 30). A process is 'primitive,' in both cases, if it greatly distorts reality for wishful or defensive purposes. It is primitive, that is, if it enables the subject to distort the world in the manner shared, in Freud's account, by primitive man and modern children. Over time any reference to Freud's phylogenetic narrative drops out. Yet the *term* primitive, which preserves the story, persists as a technical word in an ostensibly neutral lexicon.

To the extent that *primary process*, *splitting* and *projective identification* remain central in the psychoanalytic lexicon, Freud's primitive man is still at play in our clinical imagination. It is important to reconsider Freud's phylogenetic perspective, not just for its own sake, but also, and more importantly, for its implicit effect on current developmental theory.

Three Obstacles

Freud's phylogenetic hypotheses and their metapsychological derivatives run into three obstacles: (1) the established rejection of Haeckel's recapitulation theory (Gould, 1977); (2) the mistaken assumption that the West's scientific/technological achievements indicate the superior rational faculties of the Western individual (Boas, 1928; Gertz, 1973); and (3), within psychoanalysis, the deconstruction of the analyst's cultural authority (Hoffman, 1983; Aron, 1991; Altman, 1993, 2000; Stern, 2003a; Brickman, 2003).

To begin, Gould (1977) has traced the Haeckelian threads implicit in Freud's phylogeny-ontogeny comparison. Cardinal among them is the assumption that the *adult* primitive is manifest in civilized *child* psychology and, by extension, in *regressive* neurotic psychology. Thus, the adult primitive killed his father and felt remorse; today's five-year-old, by contrast, undergoes the Oedipus complex. Gould demonstrates that research in evolutionary biology—beginning, in fact, before Haeckel with von Baer (1828)—has not supported the adult-ancestor/child-descendent equation.

Gould (1977) proposes, with von Baer, that, "the vast majority of supposed recapitulations represent nothing but the conservative nature of heredity" (p. 4). This alternative recognizes that, as von Baer pointed out, many features of embryos in higher animals are not present in lower adult animals. The placenta, for instance, is an adaptation to uterine life. There is no ancestral adult precursor. "No adult ancestor," as Gould (1977) puts it, "could have lived in an artificial pond created by its own skin" (p. 163).

Gould's critique of psychoanalysis is limited to an exposé of the Haeckelian assumptions in Freud's ontogeny–phylogeny comparison. His comments are meant not as a primary critique of psychoanalysis but as part of a broader effort to demonstrate the social impact of Haeckelian thought. The implication for psychoanalysis, which leads beyond Gould's project, is that, by questioning Haeckel's position, we cast doubt on Freud's phylogenetic claims. It is left for psychoanalysis to determine, on the basis of its own methods, if the problems in Haeckel indeed undermine the Haeckel-inspired pillars of Freud's conceptual edifice.

To be precise, Freud did not argue that civilized man transcends primitive psychology. He argued specifically that civilized man sublates his primitive feeling of omnipotence into a practical and scientific effort to satisfy his wishes in the external world. The capacity for scientific thought thus becomes an index of psychological development.

This point leads into the second obstacle—treating scientific achievement as an index of psychological capacity. Such a link mistakenly takes the West's scientific achievements as a sign of its people's innately superior capacity for rational adaptive thought. The consequence is devastating. Individuals who lack the cultural resources of a Western education are considered deficient in their innate capacity for secondary process. Against this view, Gertz (1973) proposes that people reason in terms of their cultural resources. The cultural material of secondary process thought—and, more specifically, the scientific and technological resources—will differ between groups. That one group lacks such resources does not mean its people have less potential for rational thought.

A broader epistemological problem, which Boas (1928) highlights, is that, while we can recognize scientific/technological progress from one generation to the next, it is impossible to bring other aspects of cultural life into an overarching progressive sequence. To attempt any such narrative is to run immediately into a conflict of ideals: "Changes that appear to one [culture] as progress appear to another as retrogression. . . . What is desirable depends upon valuations that are not universally accepted" (p. 202). If we cannot establish a line of cultural progress, beyond scientific and technological advances, then the story line of man's more general evolution, of which it was the index, is left without support.

The critique of Freud's phylogenetic/ontogenetic narrative leads, however, beyond the problems raised in evolutionary biology and cultural anthropology. The "figure of the primitive" (Brickman, 2003) endures perhaps less out of any studied devotion to Freud's phylogenetic claims than out of a fantasy: the analyst as an intrepid explorer and colonizer of untamed lands.

Here we arrive at the third obstacle: the deconstruction of the analyst's cultural authority. As early as 1968, Racker critiqued the 'myth' that "analysis is an interaction between a sick person and a healthy one" (p. 130). The analyst, like the patient, is a conflicted person who contributes to the analytic situation in ways that he—because of his own defenses—does not see. Building on this point, Hoffman (1983) argued that the patient makes plausible inferences about conscious and unconscious tendencies in the analyst. The implication, which Aron (1991) fleshes out, is that a thorough analysis must include the analysis of the patient's experience of the analyst's subjectivity—not just to sort out the patient's projections onto the analyst, but to recognize the patient's potential for genuine insight into how unconscious tensions in the analyst might influence their relationship.

Stern (2003a) brings the issue of prejudice (e.g., cultural prejudice) to bear on the question of the analyst's unconscious contribution to the analytic dialogue. By *prejudice* he means, following Gadamer (1960), the biases or expectations we develop both through our own personal history and through our constant immersion in overlapping cultural traditions. Such prejudices, or biases, both facilitate and obstruct our understanding of others. To explore the analyst's unconscious participation is in part, then, to explore the cultural prejudices by which he might misread the analysand's experience. The prejudice of Western superiority is one such example. It works unconsciously, by force of tradition, to suggest that the analyst is more rational—indeed more evolved—than his primitive patient.

It takes courage to recognize, let alone publish on, feelings of cultural superiority in the countertransference. Altman (1993, 2000) has presented several cases in which African American patients of low socioeconomic status showed difficulty tolerating anxiety in the analytic situation, a focus on concrete help and a tendency to communicate intense affect through nonverbal action (e.g., missed sessions and nonpayment). One patient, Linda, was hospitalized by her sister after losing her temper and throwing dishes at her boyfriend. Several times in the past she had received pills for her 'nerves,' which she took irregularly, no matter how they were prescribed. This time a psychology intern spoke to her at length. The intern heard a long history of betrayals by parents and lovers, and linked them to the patient's current suspicion of her boyfriend's infidelity. The patient said that talking was helpful and left the clinic without asking for medication. To the intern's disappointment, though, Linda did not show up for their next session. Since Linda had no phone, the intern wrote her a letter. For two weeks there was no response. In the third week, Linda showed up unscheduled to ask the intern to send her medical records to the Social Service Administration. She hoped to obtain financial assistance from the government for people who cannot work due to a physical or mental disability. The therapist felt confused, irritated and ambivalent. She did not want to reject what might have been a legitimate request but, on the other hand, felt that to comply might be to collude with what seemed a hostile, exploitative and despairing position. The case history lacks the sustained immersion needed, in my view, to support a convincing conceptualization. It does, however, suggest how easy it might be for the therapist to blame the patient's disorienting behavior on her primitive constitution. It is evident, nonetheless, that the patient's despairing actions reflect not the condition of prehistoric humanity, but a complex adaptation to poverty and betrayal in a major international city.

The patient–analyst relationship is asymmetrical by design (Aron, 1991; Modell, 1991; Hoffman, 1991, 1992, 1994). The analyst assumes responsibility for facilitating an analytic process focused on the patient. The patient, in turn, is expected to be more emotionally vulnerable. It is inevitable that cultural prejudices, mired in implicit social power structures, will play out within their asymmetrical bond. The task of analysis, as a hermeneutic discipline, is not to deconstruct one's implicit cultural biases into nonexistence—a prejudice against prejudice (Gadamer, 1960)—but to recognize the unexpected ways in which one's prejudices manifest and disrupt open-minded analytic inquiry. The figure of the primitive is helpful, from this perspective, not as a literal concept but as the recognizable expression of a perhaps common countertransference fantasy.

Primitive ≠ Primary

The *Oxford English Dictionary* defines 'primitive' as "relating to, denoting, or preserving the character of an early stage in the evolutionary or historical development of something." To save the term—in its psychoanalytic sense—one might reject its evolutionary, or phylogenetic, meaning and narrow the term to refer strictly to individual development. It would then designate simply the *earliest*, or *primary*, forms of infantile thought.

This strategy finds some support in Freud's "Formulations on the Two Principles of Mental Functioning." There Freud (1911) asserts that in earliest infancy, the 'primary processes' are the "only kind of mental processes" (p. 218). The primary processes strive to obtain pleasure by 'hallucinatory' means. Only when hallucination fails to satisfy is the infant forced to recognize and adapt to external reality. In this account, there is no mention of phylogenetic heritage; it is arguably irrelevant to Freud's claim about infancy.

The question, then, is whether primitive psychology is truly primary in infantile development. By *primary* we mean an original state. Primary narcissism, for instance, is the first manifestation of ego-libido (Freud, 1914). Primary masochism is masochism without a cause (Freud, 1920). The problem is that, by this standard, hallucinatory wish fulfillment, the principal operation of the primitive mind, does *not* appear to be primary.

Freud (1900) implicitly recognized its non-primacy in his description of the hungry baby:

> A hungry baby screams or kicks helplessly. But the situation remains unaltered, for the excitation arising from an internal need is not due to a force producing a *momentary* impact but one which is in continuous operation. A change can only come about if in some way or other (in the case of the baby, through outside help) an 'experience of satisfaction' can be achieved which puts an end to the internal stimulus. An essential component of this experience of satisfaction is a particular perception (that of nourishment, in our example) the mnemic image of which remains associated thenceforward with the memory trace of the excitation produced by the need. As a result of the link that has

> been thus established, next time this need arises a psychical impulse will at once emerge which will seek to re-cathect the mnemic image of the perception and to re-evoke the perception itself, that is to say, to re-establish the situation of the original satisfaction. An impulse of this kind is what we call a wish; the reappearance of the perception is the fulfilment of the wish; and the shortest path to the fulfilment of the wish is a path leading direct from the excitation produced by the need to a complete cathexis of the perception. Nothing prevents us from assuming that there was a primitive state of the psychical apparatus in which this path was actually traversed, that is, in which wish ended in hallucinating. Thus the aim of this first psychical activity was to produce a 'perceptual identity'—a repetition of the perception which was linked with the satisfaction of the need.
>
> (pp. 564–565)

The infant registers a real (nonhallucinatory) internal need: hunger. He screams or kicks. The actual (nonhallucinatory) mother or caregiver provides an actual breast or bottle. The infant forms a memory trace, or mnemic image, of the real experience of nourishment. The next time the need arises, he evokes the memory trace of the original feed. The hallucinatory breast is thus a secondary, or derivative, phenomenon. The hallucinatory aim is to produce a 'perceptual identity' with the template of an actual past experience.

Freud (1911) later omitted the actual event that forges a template for hallucinatory gratification. He tacitly acknowledged, though, that it is impossible *not* to assume such a precedent:

> I shall be returning to lines of thought which I have developed elsewhere when I suggest that the state of psychical rest was originally disturbed by the peremptory demands of internal needs. When this has happened, whatever was thought of (wished for) was simply presented in a hallucinatory manner, just as still happens to-day with our dream-thoughts every night. It was only the non-occurrence of the expected satisfaction, the disappointment experienced, that led to the abandonment of this attempt at satisfaction by means of hallucination.
>
> (p. 218)

> It will rightly be objected that an organization which was a slave to the pleasure principle and neglected the reality of the external world

> could not maintain itself alive for the shortest time, so that it could not have come into existence at all. The employment of a fiction like this is, however, justified when one considers that the infant—provided one includes with it the care it receives from its mother—does almost realize a psychical system of this kind.
>
> (p. 218, n. 4)

The first passage jumps from the internal need over the original real feed, which appeared in his 1900 statement, to the hallucinatory gratification. The second passage, a footnote, admits that no organism could survive on hallucinatory gratification absent real material nourishment. Freud suggested that the 'fiction' of the infant's solipsism is justified because the infant 'almost' realizes a self-contained state in his nondifferentiation from the mother. The qualifiers are essential because they recognize a primary reality principle that operates before, and in fact makes possible, the activation of derivative hallucinations.

This is not a new critique. There is, in fact, a long tradition of theorists and researchers who have argued, in one form or another, for the primacy of the reality principle. Hartmann (1939) argued that a basic reality-orientation is prerequisite to and constitutive of the child's earliest libidinal desires. The pursuit of solipsistic pleasure cannot explain, as he points out, why certain highly adaptive modes of behavior—e.g., nursing—are endowed with greater 'pleasure potentialities' than other modes. "The libidinal activity of the oral zone leans," for example, "upon the alimentary need" (p. 44). Hartmann suggests that the capacity to tolerate frustration and anticipate the future—what Freud (1911) meant by the reality principle—develops with experience. The child develops not from pleasure to reality, then, but from immature to mature reality-orientation.

Fairbairn (1952) later arrived, though from a different direction, at a similar conclusion. He argued that since there can be no wish without a wishing subject, we must regard libidinal impulses, from earliest infancy, as the expression of ego structures. "Impulses are but the dynamic aspect of endopsychic structures and cannot be said to exist in the absence of such structures" (p. 88). If the ego, by definition, serves a reality-oriented adaptive function, and some rudimentary ego is implicit in the infant's earliest impulsive activity, then it follows that from the beginning of life, the infant is reality-oriented. "What the child lacks," Fairbairn concludes, "is experience of reality; and it is this, rather than any lack of orientation to reality, that gives the adult observer the impression that the child's behavior is primarily determined by a pleasure principle" (p. 140).

Lear (1998) has more recently framed the movement from primary to secondary process, not as an advance from hallucination to reality, but as a progression from infantile to mature thought. The infant, he writes, is "directed to the world from the beginning of mental life" (p. 84). Without this assumption we cannot explain how the infant learns to hallucinate the breast in the first place. The concrete images of primary process (e.g., the hallucinated breast) are "proto-conceptual": "They are *that from which* concepts emerge" (p. 85). The fantasy breast, in this revision, "is not the satisfaction of the wish so much as an expression of the content of the wish. It is what the wish is for" (p. 78). The infant begins, then, in Lear's Freudian revision, with a primary reality-orientation.

This theoretical trend accords with psychoanalytic infant observation. Stern (1985) synthesized an array of findings in infant observation to demonstrate that the "infant engages in the same kind of active regulatory traffic with the external world as does anyone at any age" (p. 233). One-month-old infants, for example, can recognize facial animation, complexity and configuration (Sherrod, 1981). They act differently in response to facial patterns than to inanimate geometric forms (Donee, 1973). The observational evidence thus supports the notion of the infant's primary orientation to reality.

The Boston Change Process Study Group (2007) go so far as to argue that real interactive processes (e.g., implicit relational knowing) constitute the bedrock of experience. Intrapsychic processes such as conflict, defense and fantasy are seen, in their model of the mind, as derivative phenomena. Their model upends the classical psychoanalytic hierarchy in which the 'interactive level' is considered derivative of deeper forces on the 'intrapsychic level' (p. 843).

An alternative position is that the two 'levels' interpenetrate each other from the beginning. The infant's *intrapsychic* wishes (e.g., to be close to his mother) color his veridical perception of *interactive* reality (Erreich, 2003). Fantasy always occurs, as Erreich elaborates, at the intersection of wishful thinking and the perception of the real environment. The effort to parse reality from fantasy—when they are always, in fact, intertwined—reflects an interpretive, or hermeneutic, problem that might arise in clinical practice. Consider, for example, the patient who feels the analyst has acted seductively toward her. She might press the analyst to recognize the reality of his flirtatious behavior instead of merely interpreting her perception as the product of her wishful projection. To explore the issue is to enter into a fluid interpretive process (Rizzolo, 2014). It is fluid because the intrapsychic (e.g., what I wish for) and the interactive (e.g., what you are really doing) are themselves fluid constructs and can never be fully disentangled.

The infant develops, then, not from an initial state of hallucinatory wish fulfillment to the reality principle, but from an immature/inexperienced reality-orientation to a mature/experienced reality-orientation. The point, for my purposes, is that the infant is reality-oriented—though in an immature way—from the beginning. Hallucinatory wish fulfillment—the defining operation of the primitive mind in Freud's theory—is not a primary operation, but a derivative one. It presupposes that the infant has already experienced and remembered a real (nonhallucinatory) satisfaction, such as that at the actual breast.

The Lifelong Development of 'Primitive' Mechanisms

One might, as a second resort, loosen the concept of primitivity. Perhaps it should refer not to an original condition of thought but, more generally, to mental patterns and operations that emerge in infancy (even if hallucination is secondary) and persist unchanged in the unconscious. One might concede, for instance, that the hallucinatory breast is a secondary phenomenon, and yet maintain that the primary processes and primitive defenses—as observed in the analyst's consulting room—are still characteristic of infantile mentation. The term *primitive* then becomes a synonym for *infantile*. It is assumed that such infantile operations remain available in the adult's unconscious.

We find this kind of solution, for instance, in Lear's interpretation of Freud's developmental theory. Lear (1998) rejects the primacy of the hallucinatory breast and yet still maintains that the child grows from the 'loose associations' of primary process thinking to the more 'honed' and 'refined' links of secondary process thinking. The claim is that, even though hallucination is secondary, the young child still thinks in loose associations. The child's loose associative thinking is thought to persist in the adult unconscious. The child, in other words, thinks consciously in the way adults think unconsciously.

We find a similar solution in Hinshelwood's discussion (1991) of primitive defenses. He suggests that primitive defenses like splitting and projective identification are primitive in the sense that they characterize the earliest phases of development. It becomes irrelevant that hallucinatory gratification is a secondary phenomenon. The claim is simply that when the analysand resorts to splitting, projective identification and other primitive defenses he resorts to operations characteristic of infancy. Thus, *primitive* defense becomes synonymous with *infantile* defense.

Such a solution relies on the alleged infantile character of primary processes and primitive defenses. More recent research suggests, however, that the analysand's loose associative thinking and defensive splitting and projective operations are not characteristic of infancy. Rather, they represent mature forms of cognition that we should not telescope back onto the newborn child. We cannot, then, treat the term *primitive* as a synonym for *infantile*. We instead require a lifespan approach in which we explore how infantile operations develop into the mature forms observed in the analysis of adults.

Condensation best illustrates the lifespan development of a primary process mechanism. By *condensation* we understand the 'compression' by which our dreams can express a range of dream-thoughts in characteristically "brief, meager and laconic" images (Freud, 1900, p. 278). The compressed links are unpacked in the analysand's later associations, which, Freud holds, reveal thoughts already active in the dream formation.

The dream of the botanical monograph gives us a sense of how Freud used this concept. The monograph in this dream condenses various memories of reading and writing:

> I had written a monograph on a certain plant. The book lay before me and I was at the moment turning over a folded coloured plate. Bound up in each copy there was a dried specimen of the plant, as though it had been taken from an herbarium.
>
> (Freud, 1900, p. 168)

From the monograph image Freud associated first to his actual *paper* on the coca plant (Freud, 1884). He recalled that a colleague, Karl Koller, had pursued a suggestion in that paper to discover the anesthetic properties of cocaine. He then remembered a festschrift he had just seen in honor of the professor in whose laboratory Koller had made the discovery. He then associated to the *bookworms* in the secondary school's herbarium. Next his mind turned to the uncompleted *monograph* of the *Interpretation of Dreams*, which lay before him like the book in the dream. He recalled a letter from Fliess in which his friend wrote, "I see it lying finished before me and I see myself turning over its pages" (p. 171). He remembered wishing that he could share Fliess's optimism: "If only *I* could have seen it lying finished before me!" He then recalled that, as a medical student he had got hold of a number of *volumes* of the proceedings of medical societies and was "enthralled by their coloured plates" (p. 172). The memory of the colored plates recalled a memory from around age five in which he and his sister had destroyed a *book with colored plates*. He associated to having become a *bookworm* himself in his student years. At age seventeen, he recalled, he ran up a balance he could not pay at the *bookseller's*. He remembered his father's displeasure at the amount. He infers the dream's meaning to be: "After all, I'm the man who wrote the valuable and memorable paper (on cocaine)." The aim of the dream, then, or at least one of its aims, would seem to be a 'self-justification': an assertion of his priority in the cocaine discovery. He asserted this priority against his self-doubt (e.g., with the current manuscript) and, in memory, against his father's apparent skepticism vis-à-vis his reading habit.

The question, for our purposes, is whether it is fair to treat this kind of mental activity as a model for childhood category formation. The dream's reliance on abstract categorization suggests that it is not, in fact, a good model (Litowitz, 2007). The associations, as we have seen, bring together a range of scenes linked by the abstract concept of reading/writing. The memories concentrate, moreover, on the theme of the dreamer's ambition. The implicit category would seem to be *ambition-laden memories of reading and writing*.[4] It suggests a capacity for conceptual abstraction uncharacteristic of children, who tend, by contrast, to form experience-bound concepts based on practical activities (Carey, 1985; Nelson, 1996; Litowitz, 2007). Cognitive research on concept formation suggests a progression from experience-bound childhood categories to the abstract links in adult condensation (Rosch & Lloyd, 1978; Carey, 1985; Nelson, 1996; Litowitz, 2007). The work of condensation is thus subject to lifespan development in abstract thinking.

Like condensation, the so-called primitive defenses also increase in sophistication across the lifespan. The defenses of splitting and projective identification illustrate this process. I will rely for convenience on Hinshelwood's definition (1991) of these defenses. He defines splitting along two axes: ego vs. object and coherence vs. fragmentation:

> Klein's early work concentrated upon the objects and their vicissitudes. She showed that from extremely early in life objects are not objectively perceived and understood—in fact they are frequently given unnaturally good natures or unnaturally bad ones. Children split their objects so that parental imagos are separately endowed in their child's imaginative play with wholly good and benign qualities and intentions, or else with wholly bad ones. As a result, splitting became a term employed to describe the way in which objects come to be separated into their good aspects and their bad ones. . . . After 1946 Klein became more interested in the *splitting of the ego* [*sic*]. In particular, she described the splitting-off of aspects of the self which were feared as bad, usually with the projective invasion of them into an object. She also described the minute splitting of objects which brings with it attendant fragmentation of the ego. This latter splitting process, which gives rise to the fear of annihilation, may have an active quality to it—that is, the ego may fragment itself or it may be more passive and dependent on the presence of absence of an integrating object.
>
> (Hinshelwood, 1991, pp. 434–435)

The person, in short, can split the ego into good and bad parts. He can also split the object into good and bad parts. In a more extreme version of splitting, he can split the ego into a coherent part and a fragmented part. He can likewise split the object into a coherent part and a fragmented part. In fragmentation, to clarify, the person obliterates a feared object by breaking it into 'bits' (Hinshelwood, 1991, p. 435). The ego falls into "a corresponding number of bits." The result is an impairment in the fragmented ego function, such as a lapse in the ego's capacity to symbolize (Hinshelwood, 2008).

The Kleinian literature has produced ample clinical evidence of splitting (see recently, Feldman, 2009; Hinshelwood, 2008; Blass, 2015). The question is whether splitting is infantile per se. Developmental research suggests that it is not (Fischer, 1980; Harter, 1986; Fischer & Ayoub, 1994; Westen, 1989). It seems, on the contrary, that splitting develops, normatively or pathologically, through latency, adolescence and adulthood.

Relevant developmental studies examine children's ability to hold contradictory emotions. Harter (1986) and Fischer and Ayoub (1994), for instance, have found that four-to-five-year-olds tend to deny the co-occurrence of two feelings. A four-year-old girl, for instance, when asked if she could be happy and sad at the same time, replied, "No way! I've only got one head" (Fischer & Ayoub, 1994, p. 150). At age six to eight children could describe how one conflicting emotion might follow another: "If you were in a haunted house you'd be scared, but then you'd be happy after you got out of it" (Harter, 1986, p. 122). Between the ages of eight and twelve children could describe the co-occurrence of two emotions: "Like at a wedding, you'd feel happy that they were getting married, but sad that they were going to move away" (p. 123). A further study found that children of an average age of 10.08 could only bring opposite-valence feelings together to bear on different targets: "I was sitting in school feeling worried about all of the responsibilities of a new pet, but I was happy that I got straight A's on my report card" (Harter, 1986, p. 128). By an average age of 11.34, children were further able to bring together opposite-valence feelings toward a single object: "I was happy that I got a present but mad that it wasn't what I wanted" (p. 128).

The implication is that splitting is not infantile per se. The mental operation of splitting develops, rather, from infantile to more mature (but still rudimentary) forms in latency. In the earliest form of splitting, the child rejects the potential co-occurrence of contradictory emotion in one mind. In a slightly more advanced form, the child allows that one contradictory might follow another in time. Even after the child can hold contradictory emotions simultaneously, and thus demonstrates a rudimentary capacity for ambivalence, we might find yet another evolution in splitting: The child might hold two contradictory feelings at the same time and yet not allow one feeling state to modify the other feeling state, as, for instance, when tender feelings soften one's hostility toward a love object.

Developmental studies of adolescents suggest a jump in the capacity for abstract splitting. Adolescents increasingly regard people in terms of complex and often hidden characteristics (Harter, 1986 Fischer & Ayoub, 1994; Rosenberg, 1979; Selman & Shultz, 1990). The growth of complexity leads to an increased perception of conflict between contrasting thoughts, feelings, traits and roles in themselves and in interpersonal relationships (Harter & Monsour, 1992; Fischer & Ayoub, 1994). Monsour (1985) and Harter (1986), for example, found a sharp rise from seventh to ninth grade in the self-perception of clashing personality traits or qualities. One subject said, "I hate the fact that I get so nervous. I wish I wasn't so inhibited! The real me is talkative; I just want to be natural" (p. 144). Another said, "I really think of myself as friendly and open-armed to people, but the way the other girls act, they force me to become an introvert, even though I know I'm really not. It really bothers me and sometimes the only way to handle it is to become immune to yourself." In semi-structured interviews with a nonclinical population Broughton (1980) illustrated the adolescent's further preoccupation with intellectual splits (e.g., essence vs. appearance, inner vs. outer, reality vs. illusion, mental vs. material, existence vs. non-existence, animate vs. inanimate, thing vs. being). Adolescents rely increasingly on such abstractions to work out unconscious internal conflicts (Anna Freud, 1936). The nature of splitting in adolescence shifts, then, toward greater abstraction: Thoughts and feelings are joined and split apart in increasingly complex networks.

Fischer and Ayoub (1994) posit an increased capacity between ages eighteen and twenty-five for recognizing the simultaneous interaction of multiple (potentially split) personality variables. It is unclear whether further development in splitting represents additional cognitive advance or simply greater lived experience in the context of new tasks and conflicts. I suggest that, in either case, even after the cognitive *process* of splitting has peaked in sophistication, the *content* and *function* of adult splitting develops across the remainder of the lifespan. The capacity to yoke multiple ways of being under abstract self and other representations allows for endless permutations in what is split and why it is split.

It might be argued that the above literature pertains more directly to 'coherent' ego and object splitting than to 'fragmenting' ego and object splitting (Hinshelwood, 1991). The studies do not describe the annihilation of split-off ego/object operations. It seems inevitable, however, that splitting-as-the-annihilation-of-operations also develops across the life cycle. It must do so because it is, in essence, the negative expression of a mental operation. The potential for such negation depends on what is available to be negated. The available functions and their interrelation reflect, in turn, their lifelong development. The vicissitudes of annihilation thus reflect the vicissitudes of the life cycle.

Projective identification develops as a function of development in splitting: The more sophisticated the split-off content, the more sophisticated the projection. The earliest form of projective identification, according to

Hinshelwood (1991), reflects a mental state in which objects have motives and emotional meaning without physical qualities:

> Projective identification was defined by Klein in 1946 as the prototype of the aggressive object-relationship, representing an anal attack on an object by means of forcing *parts of the ego* into it in order to take over its contents or to control it and occurring in the paranoid schizoid position from birth. . . . It is true that the ability to get into an object and control the way it feels and responds sounds very sophisticated. It is clearly possible to perceive this occurring in both adult patients and child patients in psychoanalysis. But could such a phantasy exist at birth? The theory of unconscious phantasy would have it that the first objects are constructed as primitive interpretations of basic bodily sensations giving pain or pleasure and the object is therefore an emotional one with motivations but without physical qualities. . . . There must be some validity in the criticism that infants cannot perform their projective identifications in as sophisticated a way as adult patients. . . . The Kleinian description of projective identification as primitive has to be qualified when describing such sophisticated interpersonal maneuvering, and restricted to the primitive quality of the concreteness of the phantasies behind the subtle methods.
>
> (pp. 179, 199)

The claim, in short, is that projective identification first operates when the infant assigns motives to objects of pain/pleasure even though he cannot yet perceive their physical features. This position rebuts an historical ego psychological critique according to which projective identification requires later ego development—specifically, the capacity to perceive a self–other boundary (A. Freud, 1936; Jacobson, 1964; Mahler, 1975; Kernberg, 1976).

The problem—both with Hinshelwood's claim and with the critique it refutes—is that the infant does seem capable at birth of perceiving the other's separate physical features (Stern, 1985). The argument for an early form of projective identification cannot presuppose a pre-perceptual object world. A stronger footing might be found in the infant's neurological propensity to imitate, intuit and match affect states (Greatrex, 2002). This innate capacity syncs with the nascent capacity, which develops notably at nine to twelve months, to perceive the other's behavior as goal directed and predictable (Gergely & Watson, 1996). These infantile operations allow for the earliest conceivable projective identification.

This earliest conceivable projective identification is, nonetheless, much more rudimentary than the usual intrapsychic/interpersonal patterns Kleinians designate by the term. (Hinshelwood makes the same observation in the passage quoted above.) Feldman (2009), for example, presents the following vignette to illustrate splitting and projective identification:

> A patient, Mr. A, arrived for the first session after a holiday and I noticed that he was moving and speaking in an unusually clear and business-like fashion. He said that when he had arrived in the waiting room, he had found another man there already (he knows that I share the premises with colleagues, and had occasionally seen other patients in the waiting room). He had not seen this particular person before, and it had disconcerted him at first. He thought I might have made a mistake, and double-booked two patients. He imagined me suddenly discovering my mistake, feeling terribly embarrassed, and not knowing how to cope with the situation. He speculated that I would probably ask one of my colleagues to go to the waiting room to call one of them out, and explain the situation to him, and then I would see whoever remained.
>
> He portrayed me, in his mind, as confused, embarrassed and, moreover, unable to face the muddle I had created—I had to send someone else to deal with it on my behalf. The patient very quickly found himself in a position where he was calmly observing the situation, not even entertaining the idea that *he* might have made a mistake.
>
> (pp. 25–26)

We learn, later in the session, that Mr. A. had himself felt muddled during the analyst's vacation:

> Later in the session, it emerged that in the course of the previous week, during my absence, he had found himself getting into a terrible mess; he had lost his watch, he hadn't known what was going on, and he described a variety of other difficulties.
>
> (p. 26)

The analyst suggests that Mr. A. had split off and projected his own muddled state into the analyst:

> What dynamic mechanisms can be invoked to account for the situation that obtained at the start of the session? It seemed to me that the patient's knowledge and experience of his own state of confusion, his embarrassment about finding himself in a mess during the holiday (expressed in his loss of the watch) became projected, in his phantasy, into me. After a momentary sense of discomfort within himself, on encountering an unfamiliar person in the waiting room, he cured himself of the unwelcome and disturbing thoughts and experience, and behaved in an efficient and well-organized way, while (in his phantasy) his analyst had to summon help to rescue himself from a muddle. . . .
>
> It was evident that the material the patient was projecting into me, in his phantasy, and taking as real properties of my mind at the time, did not constitute the whole contents of his mind. He preserved a way of functioning that was well organized, and was able to work out, in quite a complex and logical fashion, how I might set about dealing with the consequences of my mistake or confusion. He even seemed sympathetic towards me. We are thus evidently dealing with a split that has taken place in his mind, making part of his mental contents temporarily unavailable to him, while colouring his perceptions and his phantasy concerning me.
>
> (pp. 26–27)

One could debate, as with any clinical material, whether the analyst's formulation is correct. I shall assume, for the purpose of discussion, that it is. We can then consider the psychological sophistication in the hypothesized splitting and projective processes. The processes described here rely, first of all, on the complex capacity to abstract a multifaceted self-representation (the 'muddled' self). The *muddled self* is confused, embarrassed and unable to face the mess he has created. He has a passive solution, moreover, for evading embarrassment: He asks someone else to take care of the mess for him. The shame and wish to save face imply a thwarted motive to do better by his patients. He is, in short, a character with conflicts, defenses and solutions. The patient splits this character off from the *calm, organized* self—an aloof character, but one apparently capable of sympathy. In his imagination the analyst comes to represent the muddled self. The patient, in turn, gets to be the calm, organized one who can sympathize with him. It is not until adolescence, as the aforementioned research would suggest, that we find the capacity to represent such a complex interaction of split self-attributes.

These complex processes rely, on an even more microscopic level, on the capacity for abstract condensation. The sense of being muddled condenses a range of muddled experiences. The patient, to be specific, feels muddled upon the analyst's departure for a vacation. It is plausible, as Hinshelwood (1991) might suggest, that the muddled state reflects traces of an early visceral pain when, as an infant, he perhaps felt the breast's absence. But any such infantile traces get linked, via condensation, with the immediate experience. He associates later in the session to colleagues who complained that he had left his office in a 'terrible mess' (p. 27). He then portrays them as "being in a mess psychologically." Potential traces of infantile pain—losing the watch—the analyst's imagined mistake—the messy office—his colleagues' being in a mess psychologically and, presumably, many experiences in between—play into the feeling of being messy in the session. Diverse forms of messiness are amalgamated in a sophisticated act of conceptual thinking.

The example suggests, then, that the operations of condensation, splitting and projective identification develop from infantile to adult forms. It follows that 'primitive' operations are not, in fact, infantile per se. They mature in the direction of increased abstraction. This, in turn, enables ongoing development in what is linked and why it is linked.

Conclusion

The concept of primitivity preserves a dated phylogenetic-ontogenetic bridge from the prehistorical subject to the third-world subject to the first-world child to the adult neurotic. The designation of 'primitive' processes as 'primitive' reflects a first-world value judgment whereby a scientific education becomes an index of the capacity for reason. A long tradition of conceptual critique, joined with recent empirical research, suggests, moreover, that many so-called primitive operations (e.g., hallucinatory wish fulfillment, condensation, splitting and projective identification) are neither primary nor infantile per se, but rather develop in conceptual sophistication across the lifespan. In discarding the term *primitive*, we discard a theoretical residue of Western prejudice and open the field of inquiry for a more accurate understanding of lifespan unconscious development.

Notes

1 First published as Rizzolo, Greg S., 'The Specter of the Primitive', 2018, *Journal of the American Psychoanalytic Association (JAPA)* 65(6): 945–977. Reprinted by permission of Sage Publications, Ltd.

2 Freud (1874, 1875) mentions Haeckel just twice in offhanded remarks in letters to his boyhood friend Eduard Silberstein. Freud was, however, as Gould (1977) notes, trained as a biologist when Haeckel's influence was prominent. He was also a self-avowed Lamarckian. In November 1917, for instance, he wrote to Karl Abraham of his idea "to put Lamarck entirely on our ground and show that his 'need,' which creates and transforms organs, is nothing but the power of Ucs ideas over one's own body, of which we see remnants in hysteria, in short, the 'omnipotence of thoughts'" (p. 360). Gould has demonstrated, to complete the link, that "recapitulation finds an almost automatic justification under Lamarckian notions of inheritance" (p. 156).

3 The savage mindset was not, however, limited to Australia. Freud (1913b) also considered the native tribes of Melanesia, Africa and the Americas to be savages.

4 The dreamer must represent the ideational content in his memories through the imagistic medium of the dream (Litowitz, 2007). The condensation process thus reflects the constraints of thinking in a picture-language. Freud (1900) considered the picture-language of dreams to be a more "primitive" medium than verbal expression (p. 547). It is difficult, however, to imagine how one might demonstrate the inherently primitive nature of imagistic thinking. An alternative would be to regard the imagistic and verbal mediums as parallel and intersecting languages—each of which develops from infantile to mature forms.

Chapter 7

The Depth of the Present

The preceding argument is often heard, in discussion with colleagues, as a reinforcement of the relatively recent and widespread interest in here-and-now process shifts. The term 'here-and-now' appears, with some overlap and some variances in usage, in post-Freudian relational theory (Gill, 1979, 1984), ego psychology (Sandler & Sandler, 1984, 1987, 1994a) and British Kleinian theory (Joseph, 1978, 1989, 2013; Blass, 2011). These writers share a common critique of the historical privilege of genetic interpretation. Such interpretation remains useful because it contextualizes the analysis of the present. The analysis of the present, however, is seen as the vehicle of therapeutic action.

By virtue of their emphasis on present interaction, here-and-now approaches are less likely than more historically focused approaches to fall into the genetic fallacies of regression logic. To the extent that they remain nested in a classical depth model of the mind, they are, however, subject to the same problems outlined in the critique of the archeological metaphor (see Chapter 2). The critique of regression therefore adds to these perspectives a clarification about the depth of the present moment. It deconstructs the idea of an unmodified infantile unconscious beneath the phenomenology of the here and now.

The depth of the present does not depend, then, on the supposed infantile nature of the repressed. It depends only on the proposition that we are guided by repressed motives and meanings. The motives and meanings themselves attest to the trajectory of the lifespan.

The dichotomy between genetic interpretation and the analysis of the here-and-now is, by implication, a false one. The former is itself a narrative expression of the present field. It reflects the psychic organization of the couple in the analytic situation. The interesting question, then, is not whether a past event happened exactly as remembered, but, rather, given the memory, what purpose/s the narration serves in the present.

The Recovery of Memory Versus the Analysis of Transference

The debate between genetic and here-and-now emphases originated in Freud's alternative emphases on the recovery of memories and the analysis of the transference neurosis. This debate emerges implicitly in the shifting emphases in Freud description of transference. Freud (1912) sometimes portrayed transference, with its pull for infantile gratification, as "the most powerful resistance" to the recovery and working through of repressed memories (p. 101). Here the analysis of transference appears a preliminary activity to the recovery of memory and reconstruction of the patient's lost infantile history. The analyst's aim is to make infantile wishes conscious and ultimately 'work through' them, a process of relinquishment and integration akin to mourning (Freud, 1917c). The emphasis, in this portrayal of the analytic process, falls on the act of genetic interpretation.

Freud (1917a) seemed, in other places, to make the analysis of transference synonymous with the process of working through. He wrote, for instance, that "our therapeutic work falls in two phases. In the first, all libido is forced from the symptoms into the transference . . . in the second, the struggle is waged around this new object and the libido is liberated from it" (p. 455). Here the transference functions not only as a resistance to remembering, but also, and more essentially, as the mechanism by which the patient's internal suffering becomes manifest and therefore accessible to analytic intervention. The act of genetic interpretation, which aims at the recovery of memory, seems, in this portrayal, to become less important than the here-and-now 'struggle' to liberate the libido from its fixation on its fantasies of gratification from its new analytic object. This struggle is waged and, in many cases, the analysis arrives at a mutually satisfactory termination with little or no recovery/reconstruction of repressed infantile memory.

The second emphasis in Freud, which privileges transference analysis, found later reinforcement in Rank, Ferenczi and Strachey's contributions the theory of therapeutic action. The patient and analyst must, according to Ferenczi and Rank (1925), resist the temptation of intellectualized, or merely theoretical, self-knowledge in their pursuit a deeper self-recognition: a more immediate, more emotionally informed, kind of self-awareness, grounded in a visceral reliving of the problems, made manifest in the analytic situation. Strachey (1934) argued, with greater specificity, that 'mutative' interpretations raise to awareness unconscious impulses at the moment in which they are directed toward the analyst. Such interpretations are mutative, he held, because they reveal to the patient the discrepancy between his harsh superego, which leads him, via projection, to expect punishment, and the relatively benign response, in the actual present, from the analyst.

One might rightly argue that Freud's vision was broad enough to encompass both genetic and transference interpretation. The above distinction, if taken too strictly, can become a false dichotomy. It is not an either/or choice, but a matter of emphasis. The proponents of the 'here-and-now' share a common preference for the latter of these emphases. The therapeutic action of analysis occurs, for them, in work with transference and, in some cases, with the manifestations of conflict outside of the room. The recovery of memory is supported by and, in turn, supports, the primary analysis of the here and now.

The Question of Depth

The contemporary discussion of the here-and-now, which includes relational, ego psychological and Kleinian perspectives, ranges across a variety of issues, the most pertinent of which, for the critique of regression, is the question of depth (or the charge of superficiality). We find it raised in the exchange between Gill, an early relationalist, and his ego psychological commentators and again between Segal and Joseph in the Kleinian school.

Gill (1979, 1984b), to begin, understood transference not as a distortion of the analytic relationship, but as an instance of selective attention, in which the patient selects from ambiguous data to construct a plausible understanding of the encounter. He focused, in particular, on the patient's sense of the analyst's contribution. While Gill did not accept the patient's understanding uncritically, he found it impossible that the analyst, as a participant in the dyad, does not make a real contribution (partly unconscious) to the transference.

If the analyst adopts this position, then the analytic inquiry begins by asking not how the patient's anxieties cause him to distort the reality of the analytic relationship, but rather, how the patient has arrived at his particular plausible construction of the interaction. The patient's (or analyst's) psychopathology is to be found not in how he distorts objective reality, but in how rigidly he insists on only certain of the potential understandings. Genetic interpretation becomes useful, in a secondary sense, in helping to see how the patient developed his unique rigidities and why he is reluctant to question them.

Ego psychological commentators, who also accept the value of transference analysis, cautioned nonetheless that too much focus on the transference, without adequate attention to the infantile past, would result in a superficial analysis. Blum (1983), for one, wrote that "a purely here-and-now approach . . . would not permit full contact with the childish fantasies and feelings which continue to excessively influence or even dominate the patient's reactions, as in transference. The childhood origin and childish character of transference would remain unexplained" (p. 596). Rangel (1981), argued similarly that, because the transference reveals only certain aspects of the neurosis, and cannot "recapitulate them in depth," the analyst must go deeper in a 'creative leap' of genetic reconstruction.

The above critique of depth remains primarily in the realm of clinical technique. The Sandlers, however, go beyond technique in an instructive metapsychological response to the issue. They posit an unconscious divided into past and present realms. The 'past unconscious,' or the 'child within,' keeps alive primitive mentation thought to have developed until around age five when Oedipal conflict necessitated the institution of repression. It never manifests directly in the analytic situation. The 'present unconscious' updates the deeper past unconscious to forge a fit with the here-and-now circumstances. The analysis of the here-and-now is thus the analysis of the present unconscious. It must be supplemented by reconstruction of events retained in the past unconscious.

The Sandler's presentation of a dual unconscious is particularly useful because, though relatively unknown, it brings into bold relief a tendency in psychoanalysis to split the internal world into deep/infantile mentation and relatively superficial/present mentation. The issue of depth is raised, here and elsewhere, as a caution against what is felt to be the potential superficiality of too exclusive a focus on the here-and-now interaction.

Joseph (1978, 1989, 2013), who seems to work independently of the above perspectives, has developed an alternative Kleinian approach to the analysis of the here-and-now. She emphasizes the analysis of transference, as does Gill, but focuses more selectively on transitions between the paranoid-schizoid and depressive positions. The patient in the paranoid-schizoid position puts unconscious pressure on the analyst to collude with the denial of persecutory anxieties, largely through pseudo-interpretations, which masquerade as insight, but, in fact, serve the aims of projective and introjective identification. The patient in the depressive position, by contrast, is better able to face his inner world and, therefore, puts relatively less pressure on the analyst, but nonetheless might draw the analyst into a defensive collusion with his defenses, for example, mania, against guilt. Psychic change proceeds, according to Joseph, through "constant minute shifts," manifest in the transference, toward and away from greater integration and responsibility. By analyzing these shifts, and the surrounding enactments, patient and analyst learn to navigate them 'less blindly' and ultimately to integrate the underlying impulses.

Joseph's emphasis on the here-and-now leads away from the privilege of genetic interpretations toward a more immediate engagement with conflicts being enacted in the moment:

> The patient may tell me that her mother was so fragile that even when she was very young she felt that she had to be very protective towards her mother. It may seem from previous experience that this refers to myself, but I suspect this is not of real use to her, nor convincing to me, unless it is being manifested in some way in the session. But it would alert me to examine, for example, whether I was talking a bit carefully, was my tone a bit delicate, etc. and if so as a consequence she might have experienced me, whether consciously or not, as pussy-footing around her rather than interpreting straight.
>
> (Joseph, 2013, p. 2)

The example illustrates how genetic material helps the analyst tune into the way in which the patient might be experiencing the present relationship. The interpretation begins there. It might then lead to the past, in order to help the patient "build a sense of [her] own continuity" and free her from her "earlier and more distorted sense of the past" (Joseph, 1985, p. 164). This act of reconstruction ideally occurs "when the heat is no longer on." The risk is that it might become a defensive evasion of the immediate encounter, which remains, even in the use of reconstruction, the main site of psychic change.

The debate between Gill and the ego-psychological theorists, who put a greater emphasis on genetic reconstruction (e.g., Rangell and Sandler), runs loosely parallel to the debate, in the Kleinian school, between Segal (1989), who, in her introduction to Joseph's work, suggests that she puts a greater emphasis than Joseph does on "the need to link the interplay in the session with the infantile context" (p. ix). Segal, in her classic paper on therapeutic action, emphasized that "the deeper the layers of the unconscious reached, the richer and the more stable the therapeutic result" (p. 212). As in ego psychology, the implicit claim in this statement is that depth is synonymous with infantile phantasy life. The differences lie mainly in disagreement about what the phantasies are, and, from a metapsychological stance, in the background theory of forces that animate them.

The Narration of the Past

The question, then, is, To what extent does the critique of regression reiterate former emphases on the here-and-now and to what extent does it clarify or add to the here-and-now discussion? I argue that it clarifies the discussion by ruling out the idea of a depth that is somehow deeper than and relatively immune to the developments of the present.

The critique of regression relies on a deconstruction of the archeological model of the mind (see Chapter 2). It becomes untenable, if one accepts this deconstruction, to parse the unconscious into a deep level of unmodified infantile mentation and a more superficial level of derivative present mentation. The psychic traces of past mentation persevere in the mind, not beneath newer levels, but through integration into present mentation.

The notion of a linear causal chain from deep unmodified infantile wishes and anxieties to more superficial manifestations in the here-and-now interaction is thus considered inaccurate. Rather, the person's deepest phantasies guide his participation in the present field and, in a circular causality, are there reconfigured, prior to explicit interpretation. The potential critique of a depth beneath the present is thus rendered obsolete.

To reconstruct the past is, it follows, to narrate *a* past from the vantage point of the here and now (Schafer, 1982). The subject, wrapped up in the phantasies and anxieties of the here-and-now, selects unconsciously from among a "plenitude of possible details" from the past, works them over internally, amplifying this, minimizing that, in order to serve some aims (e.g., the impulse to disparage a past figure) and to reject other trends (e.g., the tendency to revive, in memory, a more vulnerable longing for the hated person).

The shifts in the here-and-now, described by Joseph, through a Kleinian lens, are to be seen partly in the shifting function of the analysand's narrative of the past. The narrative might, for instance, serve the aim of evasion through paranoid-schizoid mechanisms. The figures of the past will then become containers for split off, projected mentation. It might, alternatively, reflect a shift toward greater integration and responsibility in the depressive position. The figures of the past—including the self—will appear in more complex ways, acting out of more nuanced motives, with agency and concern.

The critique of regression broadens the Kleinian view by reframing all regressive fixations as here-and-now configurations. We find a complex field interaction between them all. It is less important to develop a comprehensive typology of positions or modes than to describe with personal specificity the ever-shifting configuration of needs, wishes, anxieties, defenses and solutions characteristic of the patient in the present moment. It is assumed that different organizations will overlap and interact in an ongoing flux of activity. The flux will register, in part, in shifts in how the analytic couple narrates the past.

An implicit assumption is that each major school of thought can, in principle, account in its own way for the mental configurations portrayed the other major schools of thought. We find, for instance, Balintian and Kohutian accounts of the paranoid-schizoid and depressive positions (Balint, 1965; Kohut, 1977). The analyst's framework will influence the way in which he understands his patient's internal world but, if he is willing to revise his perspective in light of Chapters 4, 5 and 6, will not undermine the fundamental critique of regression.

It is important to emphasize that the patient narrates the past in the context of a present field in which he has already been influenced by—and is responding to—the analyst's participation (Stern, 2010, 2015). The way in which he both unconsciously recalls and consciously organizes the past reflects and makes a new move in the analytic interaction. His remembrance, for instance, of an inconsistent and narcissistic mother might spurn the analyst, who seems to insist on his own benevolence, into a tacit concession that mothers—and figures like him—often fail to live up to their implicit promises.

The distinction between narrative and historical truth (Spence, 1982) has, I believe, been misunderstood, or misused, to suggest that what is at stake is a contest between the pursuit of true causal effective history and the construction of convenient fictions. What is at stake, rather, is the question of how one constructs the efficacy of the past. In doing so, one automatically selects not between truth and falsehood, but between different ways of understanding one's past with more or less equivalent empirical plausibility. To complicate matters, the construction itself and the field of which it is an emergent product work to develop the historical efficacy of the very past events in question. That is to say, the true historical efficacy of the past is itself a constant work in progress.

It is helpful to revisit Ferro's distinction between three vertices of clinical interest: the Freudian focus on the actual past, the Kleinian focus on the internal object, and the Bionian focus on transformations in the here-and-now relational field. The contribution of the critique of regression to the discussion of the here-and-now is to suggest that these are not discrete vertices in which the traces of the first two somehow lie deeper than workings of the third. It suggests, rather, that transformations in field reconfigure all layers of depth, modifying internal objects, thereby developing the efficacy of the actual past.

Chapter 8

The Case of John

A metapsychological revision should have implications for how we listen to clinical process. The central implication of the regression critique is that one ought to listen not only for resonances with the past, but also for novelty in the context of the present. The final two chapters explore this shift in attention, first in the case history of what the analyst deemed a defensive regression, second in the report of a restorative regression.

The first step, before getting into process material, is to outline the guiding methodology. I argue for a hermeneutic approach. It impossible to falsify entire regression theories. A proponent of regression can always argue that the ostensibly falsifying evidence screens a latent unconscious level on which regression hypotheses are valid. It is possible, however, to show that the prejudices of regression theory lead us to erroneous expectations, which, in turn, obscure a more complete lifespan account of the process. The suggestion is that, since completeness is an inherent good, one ought to abandon regression prejudices for a lifespan appreciation of novelty in the context of repetition.

The case of John, to continue, presents what the analyst considers a defensive regression from a dangerous internal Oedipal situation to an anal phase fixation (Haft, 2005). The anal fixation is posited to account for the emergence of John's obsessional symptoms. He thus finds himself burdened with the imperative to neutralize perceived contaminants (among other messy hazards) in a symbolic effort to manage his anal sado-erotism.

The interpretation rests on the theory that obsessional neurosis, in general, reflects a regression from Oedipal castration anxiety to an anal fixation (Freud, 1908, 1909, 1913a, 1917a, 1917b, 1923, 1926; Jones, 1918; Abraham, 1923, 1924; Shengold, 1985). The theory leads us to expect a specific causal narrative: a shift from uniquely phallic-genital phase wishes/anxieties to uniquely anal phase wishes/anxieties will yield obsessive-compulsive symptoms.

The clinical process, without falsifying the theory, calls the causal narrative into question. It does, in fact, capture something of the patient's use of obsessional defenses against destructive impulses. The destructive impulses do not, however, seem uniquely anal in character. It becomes evident, without dismissing potential anal-phase causes, that we need a lifespan history to understand the patients experience and fear of his own aggression.

The idea of the patient as an anal toddler becomes, in turn, a field character instead of a literal attribution. The patient, it is argued, invites the analyst to regard him as such in the transformation of passive castration fears into the active enactment of self-emasculation. It is less important to defend the implied correlation of this character with his actual toddlerhood than it is to explore the enactment in the immediate intersubjective field.

Method

A comparative analysis of this nature implicitly involves complex epistemological problems. Following Popper (1935) and Grunbaum (1984), Hinshelwood (2013) argues that, in comparative case study research, each side must present a 'risky' hypothesis: a hypothesis that makes a prediction, which can, in turn, be verified or falsified in the analytic process. The assumption is that the psychoanalytic situation is, in the ideal, a neutral setting, free of theoretical biases, which might color how one interprets the findings.

The greatest epistemological problem in the critique of regression is, however, that regression theories rely on the imagery of an infantile unconscious beneath the empirical process. The hypotheses they suggest are therefore *unrisky*. Whatever happens in the observable process, one can argue (as the Sandlers illustrate) that it is reflective of present unconscious updates, and that, beneath these superficialities, there lies a deep layer of truly regressive mentation, which, to reiterate, can only be reconstructed via theory.

I have addressed the vicious nature of this hermeneutic circle in Chapter 2. A hermeneutic epistemology can, I believe, lead us out of this circle into a more generative one. Such an epistemology can make use of

Hinshelwood's model by re-defining *risk* to mean not *capable of falsification*, but *capable of being questioned* in light of empirical experience. The search for neutral falsification is replaced by a search for the anomalous: an event that deviates from expectations (Khun, 1962) and therefore calls the theory into question.

The guiding aim is to remain open to questioning one's own prejudices in light of experience (Gadamer, 1960). A generative hermeneutic circle emerges between the analyst's theory and the empirical process (Rizzolo, 2014). The ideal of prejudice-free neutrality is replaced with the ideal of open-mindedness nested in perpetual unanalyzed bias.

For practical purposes, then, I have replaced Hinshelwood's terms *prediction* and *falsification* with the terms *expectation* and *confirmation/disconfirmation*. Although neutral prediction and falsification are impossible aims, the analyst's theory does lead to certain expectations, capable of articulation, which the clinical process can confirm or disconfirm. The aim is not a neutral conclusion, but the process itself of grappling with a prejudice.

Hinshelwood (2008) argues that predictions can be stated in the form of *questions*, which, in turn, can be falsified by the clinical process. I suggest similarly that the analyst's expectations can be formulated as questions capable of (dis)confirmation in the process. The question thus mediates between the expectation and empirical clinical data.

The best case for the critique of regression, then, is not to disprove what cannot be disproven. It is, rather, to highlight a bias toward the infantile, which, in spite of its potential heuristic value, might obscure relevant questions about later development in the field.

The Anal Organization

Freud (1913a, 1917b, 1923, 1926) considered the symptoms of the obsessional neurosis to be the result of a regression (to evade castration) from the genital to the anal organization. Dangerous genital strivings were replaced by erotic-sadistic impulses to evacuate, on the one hand, and on the other hand, to retain and control the object-as-feces.

The obsessional neurotic, who had regressed to anality, was noted to be orderly, parsimonious and obstinate (Freud, 1908). The trait of orderliness referred, in Freud's usage, to a preoccupation with cleanliness and a conscientiousness in carrying out small duties. By parsimony, he mean a resistance to using or spending resources, which could transform, under unspecified conditions, into more miserly manifestations of greed or avarice. Obstinacy, by contrast, indicated a stubbornness that could morph into defiance or rage.

Freud (1908) understood these three traits as reactions against/sublimations of an interest in feces. Orderliness seemed to be "a reaction formation against an interest in what is unclean and disturbing and should not be part of the body," first and foremost, feces (p. 171). The pleasure in hoarding seemed the residue of an original pleasure in holding back stool. To be obstinate seemed a residue of his self-will in parting with his excrement.

Behind these traits, Freud found side-by-side expressions of anal erotism and anal sadism. The underlying anal erotism could be parsed into active and passive aims (Freud, 1905, 1913, 1917a, 1917b). The active aim appeared in the instinct for mastery, that is, mastery of the sphincter; the passive aim in the wish to be penetrated anally and thus in homoerotic trends. The sadistic component manifested, in a complimentary fashion, in the wish to dominate or, alternatively, to destroy by evacuation (see Jones, 1918; Abraham, 1923, 1924).

The typical obsessional neurotic, Freud held, concealed his erotic and loving impulses behind more manifest, but still resisted, eruptions of sadistic or violent impulses:

> In obsessional neurosis . . . it is the regression of the libido to the preliminary stage of the sadistic-anal organization that is the most striking fact and the one which is decisive for what is manifested in symptoms. The love-impulsion is obliged, when this has happened, to disguise itself as a sadistic impulsion. The obsessional idea "I should like to kill you" . . . means at bottom nothing other than "I should like to enjoy you in love."
>
> (Freud, 1917b, p. 343)

The idea "I should like to kill you," to be consistent, should find symbolic expression not in a phallic register, but in an anal one, for example, evacuation or anal penetration. The latent erotic impulse should also emerge, if we are to be consistent with the hypothesis of an anal regression, in an anal register, for example, the wish to be penetrated anally. The sadistic-erotic duality is exemplified in the Rat Man's fear of anal torture: "While he was telling his story his face took on a very strange, composite expression. I could only interpret it as one *of horror at pleasure of his own of which he himself was unaware*" (Freud, 1909, p. 166).

The obsessional's hate, perhaps closer to consciousness than his love, is nonetheless rejected, in Freud's theory, by the superego and repressed in the dynamic unconscious:

> We may regard the repression of [the Rat Man's] infantile hatred of his father as the event which brought his whole subsequent career under the dominion of the neurosis.
>
> (Freud, 1909, p. 237)

And,

> Not only will the early aggressive impulses be re-awakened [in puberty]; but a greater or lesser proportion of new libidinal impulses—in bad cases the whole of them—will have to follow the course prescribed for them by regression and will emerge as aggressive and destructive tendencies. In consequence of the erotic trends being disguised in this way and owing to the powerful reaction-formations in the ego, the struggle against sexuality will henceforward be carried on under the banner of ethical principles. The ego will recoil with astonishment from promptings to cruelty and violence which enter consciousness from the id, and it has no notion that in them it is combating erotic wishes, including some to which it would not otherwise have taken exception. The overstrict super-ego insists all the more strongly on the suppression of sexuality, since this has assumed such repellent forms. . . .
>
> A good deal of what has been said may be objected to on the ground that the unpleasant obsessive ideas are themselves quite conscious. But there is no doubt that before becoming conscious they have been through the process of repression. In most of them the actual wording of the aggressive instinctual impulse is altogether unknown to the ego, and it requires a good deal of analytic work to make it conscious. What does penetrate into consciousness is usually only a distorted substitute which is either of a vague, dream-like and indeterminate nature or so travestied as to be unrecognizable.
>
> (Freud, 1926, pp. 115–116)

The libido regresses, then, from the phallic-genital to the anal organization and assumes the form of a sadistic impulse. The sadistic impulse is, in turn, repressed. It emerges in substitute ideas, which, like manifest dream images, are vague enough to escape moral censorship.

Freud's (1926) portrayal of the superego in obsessional neurosis complicated the picture of regression. He held the fear of the superego to be a strong determinant of the obsessional's anxiety. The fear of the superego, in turn, was associated with latency: It presupposed a passage from castration anxiety in the phallic phase through the Oedipus complex to the internalization of the parental prohibition against the child's sexual possession of the mother. It would seem to negate the idea of a total regression to the pre-Oedipal anal phase, where, in Freud's developmental theory, the danger of loss is most dominant. We can clarify the situation if we assume, with Ferenczi and Rank (1925), that the superego can regress from its post-Oedipal state to a precursor state of 'sphincter morality,' in which the prohibition is not yet against genital wishes, but against making a mess.

A series of later contributors elaborated on the Freudian theory of anal regression. Jones (1918), one of the earliest such contributors, differentiated between an interest in the anal canal and an interest in feces. The former could lead, he suggested, to a preoccupation with the "reverse side of things and situations": the back side of objects and places, a proneness to reverse words and letters in writing, a fascination for underground passages, canals and tunnels, a wish to get to the center of places and ideas etc. (p. 423). The latter could lead, by contrast, to a preoccupation with feces symbols: dirty objects, other bodily excretions, contaminants, money, children and so on (pp. 424–427).

Abraham (1923, 1924) further divided the anal phase into two sub-phases. In the first sub-phase, the child is preoccupied with pleasurable and sadistic experiences of evacuation. In the second sub-phase, when he has attained greater sphincter control, the child becomes more centrally preoccupied with conserving, retaining and controlling his objects.

Shengold (1985), who, in turn, elaborates on Abraham, suggests that the attainment of sphincter control in the second anal sub-phase facilitates the 'anal birth' of the self:

> In the second anal phase, the sphincter becomes an instrument which also is used to hold on with and to contain. The registration of the

> transient experience of the anus holding on and closing down makes the registration of a close system possible; the child can know what it is like to feel his body as an entity with boundaries and with doors that shut.
>
> (Shengold, 1985, p. 51)

> What I have been outlining amounts to the metaphoric view of the psychological birth of the human being as an 'anal birth.'
>
> (Shengold, 1985, p. 52)

The attainment of sphincter control thus allows the differentiation, or birth, of a bounded self. The implication is that, should problems occur in the phase, or should the person regress to the anal organization, he might falter in his differentiation between inside and outside.

Expectations

The theoretical discussion above leads to the following regression-specific expectations:

1. There will be a decrease in phallic-genital wishes/anxieties and an increase in anal wishes/anxieties.
2. The shift from a predominantly phallic-genital organization to a predominantly anal organization will lead to a rise in obsessive-compulsive symptoms and behaviors.
3. The structure and content of the anal wishes/dangers will be unique to the anal phase.

Questions

The expectation lead, in turn, to the following questions:

1. Is there a decrease in phallic-genital wishes/dangers, manifest, for instance, in less prominent representation of genital penetration and/or punishment for genital striving? And is there a correlated increase in anal wishes/anxieties, manifest, for instance, in more imagery of retention/evacuation, or an increased fear of making a mess?

2. Does the above transformation, if it occurs, lead to a rise in obsessive-compulsive symptoms/behaviors, manifest, for instance, in an increased preoccupation with cleanliness.
3. Are the structure and content of the anal wishes unique to the anal phase, manifest, in positive terms, in the presence of features not equally characteristic of later developmental phases, and, in negative terms, in the absence of later emerging phantasies, defenses and solutions?

The Patient

John, a pleasant-mannered accountant in his forties, sought help for his terror of contamination and an ever more restrictive set of behaviors intended to manage perceived toxins. He lived in only one part of his apartment, for example, because, in the other part, there were piles of newspapers and dirty laundry that he believed to be contaminated with cat feces. He refused to discard or wash them for fear of exposing his neighbors to feline toxoplasmosis. Similar worries and avoidances permeated his daily routine. If he felt his desk had become contaminated, he would work holding his bookkeeping ledgers in mid-air. If he passed a blood-like smear on the street, or a person with irritated or scabbed skin, he would fear he had been infected and, by turns, would worry about infecting others.

Beyond contagions, John feared fire and tripping hazards. He stepped gingerly across the analyst's rug lest he disrupt it and leave her to trip. Often he had to return to the air conditioner to make sure he had not dislodged the cord or disrupted the plug in the socket.

He seemed concerned to protect himself and the analyst against intruders. He would slam the waiting room door from the inside and press it shut to be sure that it was closed.

John had also been celibate for years. He allowed himself to masturbate only to the images of women who had given him implicit permission: women in porn, or past lovers.

In the first session, John spoke with excitement of his desire to touch the analyst, describing the anatomy of the vagina "as if separate from the whole body and personality of a woman" (Haft, 2005, p. 1105). He commented on analyst's appearance and assumed religion, seemingly to degrade her, but then felt guilty and imagined himself comforting her.

The patient grew up in what the analyst implicitly portrays as a volatile Oedipal triangle: a helpless, over-stimulated child, a sadistic father and a seductive-castrating mother:

> John was reared by both parents in a rural area of the Midwest. His mother went to her job during the hours when his father was home from work, enabling the parents to share in his care. John recalled, from before age four, often seeing his parents fighting. He described coming upon them holding up kitchen chairs toward each other while he, flooded with anxiety, retreated to his room to talk to a comforting stuffed animal. He observed when a little older that his parents' fights usually began with his mother's running out of the parental bedroom, his father in pursuit. Then, while his father physically assaulted his mother, John impotently clung to her leg, unable to protect her. The next day, John's mother would show him the bruises over her arms and on her torso and say, "You should see what your father did!"
>
> When his father was away on frequent business trips, John was delighted. He would sleep in his mother's big bed, next to her. In his analysis, he retrieved the joyful memory of reading newspapers in bed with her before falling asleep—looking as though he were reading the news when he was actually looking at the comic strips.
>
> The patient also reported the memory that, at five to six years of age, he told his mother of an 'itch' he had; and, soon afterward, his pediatrician said to his mother, "We'll get him while he's sleeping." John told me that, during that conversation, his mother 'jokingly' said to the doctor, "I know he masturbates. He lies on his stomach with his hands on his penis and rocks and masturbates." The patient was then re-circumcised in a hospital, he said, "because it was not done right the first time"; he was left with permanent scars on his penis. At about age seven, he underwent a tonsillectomy.
>
> (Haft, 2005, pp. 1106–1107)[1]

John could not protect his mother against his father. During his father's trips, however, he seemed to relax and apparently delighted in playing the role of a grown man in his mother's bed. His mother seemed to like showing him her bruised body. It is unclear how John responded to her complicated overture. The passage implies that, to the extent he felt aroused, he was met with perceived castration threats from his mother and various doctors.

When John was eleven, his father died of cancer. John felt, the analyst writes, that his destructive impulses, which he had until then displaced onto his pets, had caused his father's death. In an apparent identification with the lost father, he began to fantasize about raping and killing his mother. The fantasy seemed to intensify through adolescence:

> This death reinforced the patient's feelings of omnipotence, as he clearly remembered having had an earlier death wish toward his father. He also tearfully recounted his own cruelty to a series of pets in the years before adolescence.
>
> When the patient was older and while alone in his mother's bedroom, he would masturbate on her bed, ostensibly to keep from getting his own bedding wet. He recalled adolescent fantasies of committing rape. With horror and shame, he recollected for the first time his long-repressed fantasies of begging his mother to engage in consensual sex, and, if she refused, of raping her and then murdering her to hide the crime. He had long remembered having had in adolescence a similar fantasy involving a young woman.
>
> (Haft, 2005, p. 1107)

He harnessed his lust and his destructive impulses, the passage suggests, into an exciting and horrifying father identification. He had already shown, in abusing animals, a readiness to move from thought to action. He now felt ashamed of his violent rape fantasies and might, I suggest further, have been afraid of his own potential to enact them.

During and after college, John dated and slept with a series of women. He seems to have shown a jealous temperament and a tendency to get caught up in triangular dramas:

> In front of one girlfriend, he asked another woman out on a date. Another time, he was hostilely disapproving of a girlfriend when she spent an evening away from him with a woman friend who was visiting from out of town.
>
> (Haft, 2005, p. 1107)

In the first situation, he flaunted his ability to replace one partner with another. In the second, the tables were turned: He was angered by a girlfriend's choice of her friend over him.

The nude female body could, it seemed, evoke a silent dread that he was unable to recognize:

> He repeatedly shared the prominent memory of one college girlfriend who was surprised that he should in fear upon seeing her naked body. He himself had no awareness of the fear that she witnessed in him, nor did he understand it.
>
> (Haft, 2005, p. 1107)

The analyst speculates that the incident evoked

> his latency-age memory of his mother's once teasing him in front of his father for John's coming into the bathroom 'to see' her naked in the bathtub—which might have evoked his castration anxiety upon visual possession of his mother's naked body.
>
> (Haft, 2005, p. 1107)

It might also have evoked, beyond the fear of being belittled and mocked for his sexual arousal, a fear of his retaliatory wish to force and punish an internal mother-temptress figure.

John retreated, the analyst suggests, after a brief effort at a stereotypically masculine job, into castrated work and a defensively platonic romance with an ex-girlfriend:

> John moved to a small seaside town with a seasonally changing population, where he rented a cottage. His first job there involved hauling very heavy logs off the beach, which he believed led to the injury of one of his testicles. John said, "My doctor told me, 'This testicle is dead.'" He regretted that he had masturbated the morning before the injury occurred because he imagined that masturbating, followed by physical strain, might have led to the ensuing testicular atrophy. John spoke of distress at this bodily injury, though he did not remember his reaction to the earlier surgeries, which were only vaguely recalled.
>
> (Haft, 2005, p. 1108)

Later, as an accountant,

> John was able to retain employment, although he could not advance on his jobs because he was very slow to complete projects; he repeatedly

> checked for accuracy. Although a certified public accountant, he sometimes accepted lower-level jobs as a bookkeeper or an assistant due to these challenges.
>
> (Haft, 2005, p. 1105)

> Eventually, John settled into a long-term, loving friendship with a former girlfriend and sexual partner, Betty, and they became nonsexual roommates, first in his cottage and later in a nearby city. Keeping the relationship nonsexual helped him repress his sadistic impulses toward her. Clearly, his difficulties in this long-term relationship (resolved through desexualization), his adolescent fantasies of rape and murder, and his treatment of college-era girlfriends all reflected his sadistic-erotic way of relating to women—which he had observed in his father. We can speculate that his sadism was both an identification with his father and a reaction to his bodily injuries and surgeries, events that may have been psychically represented as punishment by a dangerous father for sexual wishes.
>
> (Haft, 2005, p. 1108)

The patient perceived the death of his testicle as a consequence of masturbation. The analyst suggests that, although John did not realize it, the setback evoked the memory of his childhood surgeries, which were felt, in her view, as a punishment for lusting after his mother. He eventually retreated into inferior accounting work, which he managed obsessively, refusing unconsciously to assert his potential and so avoiding the danger of being cut down. With Betty, meanwhile, he constructed a platonic intimacy, in which he could enjoy some feeling of closeness, without awakening his disruptive sadistic-erotic impulses.

Clinical Process

The sequences below are taken from Haft's (2005) case history. She presents the clinical process in a recursive, rather than linear, style. I have taken the liberty to cull passages from her report and reorganize them to reflect a loosely linear account of the analysis.

> *Sequence 1*
>
> Crude erotic fantasies involving me, or rather me as body parts, erupted in the first hour. For example, he excitedly spoke of his desire to touch

> me sexually, describing the anatomical parts of the vagina as if separate from the whole body and personality of a woman. At the same time, his comments on my appearance and assumed religion aimed at degrading me. Deeply pained remorse (just as with Freud's Rat Man), with fantasies to comfort his emotionally wounded analyst, followed.
> (Haft, 2005, p. 1105)

In the following weeks,

> John began many sessions with an insult about my body, my attire, or my character. He also continued to tell me about his fantasies in regard to me, usually rather aggressive and at times quite violent ones. He reported these verbal and fantasized attacks with little access to angry, hurt, or vulnerable feelings; rather, he conjectured that such feelings *might* underlie such hostile images. He repeated his withering 'beauty' reviews of me, as he called these commentaries, and often reported general anti-Semitic thoughts or slurs that popped into his mind, specifically about me. After that expression of aggression, a surge of emotional warmth and protectiveness welled up within him. Then he imagined scenes of comforting me, with his arms protectively around me, "like a father holding his daughter" after she has been rejected by a beau, or of heroically rescuing me from anti-Semitic thugs. Violent images of attacking me himself with a knife or a two-by-four piece of lumber, or smashing my skull with a claw hammer, emerged without conscious anger at the times he thought of himself as most vulnerable and manipulated by me. In a frightened rush of words, he then sought to reassure me that he would never act upon these fantasies. Nevertheless, he imagined that I had manipulated him into paying me a higher fee, and, another time, that I had 'cheated' him of the full time of the session.
>
> In the main, John did continue to exude a warm friendliness toward me. He openly expressed strong, loving feelings, deep attachment, and gratitude for our relationship. He frequently reported sexual arousal and 'semen oozing' in the session. His assessment that I looked attractive was sometimes followed the next day, however, by a disclaimer that "perhaps I was just trying to be nice yesterday."
>
> One day, in an unusual ownership of *feeling* [sic], rather than his more typical report of an emotionally detached thought, John said, "I felt myself smirking at calling you 'homely'—I felt a sort of glee to

> 'get' you again." On another occasion, when I, in a moment of countertransferential disquiet, implied that he was exaggerating damage to me from his insults, John became angry at thinking that his power over me had been taken away. Though he vigilantly watched for signs of warmth from me (which he eagerly devoured), and became crushed and fearful if he did not see a welcoming smile from me, I knew—while we briefly, smilingly, faced each other when he entered the consulting room—that he would later graphically report how unattractive I had looked to him. As John's yearnings for me intensified, his sadistic impulses also intensified.
>
> (Haft, 2005, pp. 1113–1115)

John expresses an immediate sexual interest in the analyst's body. His sexual desire, which has a sadistic, objectifying quality, morphs into an impulse, which he enacts, through his 'beauty reviews' and anti-Semitic insults, to provoke and degrade her. When he feels manipulated, or cheated out of time, he becomes more aggressive, imagining himself, for instance, beating her with a board or smashing her skull with a hammer.

His impulses and actual conduct evoke unbearable guilt and a reactive surge of warmth and protectiveness. He externalizes his destructive feelings in the form of cruel lovers and thugs. He indulges in the fantasy of her as a daughter in need of his love and protection.

The patient's guilty conscience reminds the analyst of the Rat Man, who, by Freud's (1909) analysis, had regressed from an Oedipal rivalry with his father to an anal fixation. It should be noted, however, that John's fantasies are not at present anal in expression, as were the Rat Man's fantasies of anal torture (Freud, 1909, p. 166), but phallic-genital: He fixates on female genitalia and declares that semen is oozing in the sessions.

The analyst (2005) notes that, through the cycle of attraction, denigration, attack, guilt and reassurance-seeking, John appears to enact an identification with his abusive father: "He seemed to be increasingly reenacting his father's sadistic relationship to his mother" (1114).

It was a particularly frightening identification, laden with guilt and, I suggest, realistic fear, because of the fluid boundary, established over time, between thoughts and actions. John feared, the analyst asserts, that his thoughts had caused his father's death in latency. By abusing pets, and later in his callous treatment of women, he made this fear a reality: He proved to his horror (and seeming delight) that his hostile thoughts had actual force.

The initial impression, then, is not of anal sadism, but of a sadistic phallic identification with his father and a disturbingly fluid boundary from impulse to actual conduct. He reacts against the sadistic identification, and achieves a momentary triumph, in the subsequent fantasy of comforting and protecting the fragile analyst against external dangers.

Sequence 2

> Often, the patient felt that he himself was transmitting a dreaded disease from one [person] to the other. Or, some information that he gave to one party about the other, such as an address, date of birth, or a research interest, might be mishandled, causing harm. For example, when he began analysis, he feared that I would access and steal his mother's funds if I had her name and date of birth, so he avoided telling me when he celebrated her birthday. . . .
>
> Upon entering the consulting room during this phase of treatment, John usually reported having seen a bandaged, scabbed, or abraded man on his way to the appointment (e.g., "On my way here, Dr. Haft, I have to tell you that I passed a man with a scab!"). He feared that, having seen such a person, he might now somehow carry contamination from the man's open skin and transmit it to me. . . .
>
> When treatment breaks coincided with his friend Betty's trips out of town, he imagined being forced into the painful choice of praying for the survival of either Betty or me, and not being allowed to pray for both.
>
> (Haft, 2005, pp. 1108–1111)

> John often felt great distress after spending enjoyable time outdoors with Betty on Sundays. He arrived to Monday-morning sessions dreading that he might have brought a Lyme disease tick into my office from the countryside, infecting me. This upsurge of symptoms expressed his conflict over his 'disloyalty' to me in spending time with Betty, in the face of my absence over the weekend. He spent hours on Sunday evenings checking himself, examining his skin for ticks. The Lyme

> disease that I might contract would debilitate me, and it would be his fault. He could not experience his fears as fantasies *representing* sadomasochistic aims; he experienced them as *literal* dangers.
>
> (Haft, 2005, p. 1119)

> Later on, in imagining himself with other women, each potential girlfriend became a provocative figure to Betty and also to me, and John continually feared that Betty or I would retaliate. In one instance, he worried that he would bring head lice onto my couch from the children who lived next door to a new woman in his life, destroying the safety of my office for other patients. With such a risk, he suffered great agitation in thinking that he and I would have to decide he should not be coming to my office. In this fantasy, he could have this woman only if he sacrificed me; or he could have me only if he lost her.
>
> (Haft, 2005, p. 1111)

> John also imagined 'running away' with me; however, he would have a recurrent vision of being ridiculed by a man in my life for being pathetic or ridiculous, a fantasy in which the other man essentially pushed him out of the triangle.
>
> (Haft, 2005, p. 1111)

The patient's erotic desire, and, it seems, his omnipotent sense of his women's dependence on his protection, leads him into a series of love triangles in which one of his female lovers feels betrayed by his devotion to another. He repeatedly laments, and seems to enjoy, feeling torn between women who are willing to compete viciously for his affection.

He seems to feel guilty for dividing his time and affection between multiple women, manifest, for instance, in his fear of transmitting a disease from one partner to the other. He worries, for instance, that he might infect the analyst with Lyme disease from his trips with Betty. He would then be at fault for harming her and subject to her retaliation.

While he imagines passing contaminants from one women to another, and so revealing his betrayal, he also pictures himself as the protector of women against outside toxins. He reports to his analyst every real and imagined toxin he encounters on his way to meet her. The contaminants, like the imagined cruel lover, or the anti-Semitic thugs, seem to represent an externalization of the danger he brings and wishes to protect her against.

John seems to derive his sense of worth largely, if not entirely, from his imagined capacity to protect his women, including the analyst, from the danger of himself so externalized. He engages in compulsive and futile actions a never-ending performance of his valor. He spends hours checking himself for ticks, for instance, but, on his way to the office, passes another imagined contaminant, and so cannot guarantee the analyst's safety. He prays for Betty and his analyst's wellbeing, but realizes, moreover, that he cannot pray for one without betraying the other and thereby re-inscribing the triangular drama.

He labors, all the while, under the fear that a more powerful man, who seems to lurk in the shadows of the analyst's life, will show him up. He is simultaneously, then, a sadistic father, a heroic defender of women, and a little boy, soon to be exposed for his imitation of manhood, just as he used to lie in his mother's bed, "looking as though he were reading the news when he was actually looking at the comic strips" (Haft, 2005, p. 1107).

Sequence 3

> John did not function as an independent adult, in that he had long periods of unemployment during which he used his mother, Betty, and me (by paying for his analysis late) to provide financial support. In the sessions, he experienced a good deal of bowel activity (urges and flatulence). Thus he communicated to me that he was really just a dependent baby who aggression was anal and not genital. His ready politeness and eagerness to please made him seem like a little boy.
>
> (Haft, 2005, p. 1112)

> By remaining unbathed for days, he created bodily odors with which he assaulted me; he picked at the skin on his ankles or fingers until they bled before coming to some sessions and would lie down, "risking contamination of the couch," he said. He reported leaving old pizza boxes in his kitchen, attacking cockroaches, which he imagined carrying into my office.
>
> The patient's aroma, 'blood droplets,' and roaches, which he actually constructed and then imagined transporting from himself to me, created a connectedness between us, which expressed his experience of our relationship. He experienced us as emotionally connected because we would be *concretely* connected via these manufactured

> symbol equivalents. His fear that a tick from the park he had visited over a weekend while apart from me might have embedded itself in him or in his clothing—and that it might crawl off his body, off the couch, over to my chair, and up my leg, embedding itself finally in my thigh—could be understood as conveying a highly charged and romantic scene between us.
>
> (Haft, 2005, pp. 1118–1120)

The third sequence suggests a potential shift from a phallic-genital to an anal mode of organization. John, who is employed on and off, pays his analytic bill late and so implicitly becomes dependent on the analyst, along with Betty and his mother, for financial support. He often farts, moreover, and expresses the urge to defecate. Unfortunately, we do not learn what fantasies (anal or otherwise) underlie his manifest conduct. We cannot assume that manifest anal behavior signifies an unconscious anal fixation (Cf. Arlow & Brenner, 1964). It might just as readily serve other psychosexual aims. Still the analyst does read his behavior in an anal light. She tells us he acted like this to show her, "he was really just a dependent baby whose aggression was anal and not genital."

The figure of the patient as a dirty little boy can understood as a here-and-now field character. The patient, in defense against his sadistic-erotic phallic impulses, and in anticipation of being emasculated, invites the analyst—e.g., by farting, neglecting his hygiene and relying on her financially—to see him as if he were nothing but a messy child. He repeats, in this move, what seems the basis of his self-castrated intimacy with Betty.

It is implied, in light of the literature on anal regression, that we can now consider the contaminants of the patient's phantasy life as feces symbols. The material does not, however, provide independent support for this possibility, for example, associations to anal wishes/fears. It would be tautological to assume that anything messy equates de facto to feces.

It must be noted, moreover, that John's preoccupation with contaminants was manifest, before the anal shift, in more immediately phallic moments, for example, of semen oozing. The trajectory of this sequence suggests that contaminants can indeed be phallic-genital symbols. John imagines a tick crawling from his body up the analyst's leg and embedding itself in her thigh. The image is less one of defecation than of phallic-genital intrusion.

In this sequence, then, that the patient moves from the expression of sadistic and erotic phallic strivings into a self-castrated position, which allows for a limited intimacy, based on the denial of his genital phantasy life. The denial can only last for so long before his genital impulses resurface. He labors obsessively to manage various contaminants, many of which, like the tick, reflect his sense of himself as an intrusive force.

Sequence 4

> As the treatment went along, John understood a bit more about himself, and he observed, "I'm starting to get the idea of wanting to be careful to protect people from me." That important development in his thinking evolved in part from my repeated suggestions that his fears of contaminating me or failing to protect my safety were of a piece with fears of harming me with words. It had been easier for him to grasp his responsibility for insulting me than to grasp the latent aggression in fantasies of creating tripping hazards and contamination dangers in my office.
>
> (Haft, 2005, p. 1114)

> Another violent and erotic transferential fantasy erupted, which appeared to be a further sign that John's sadistic drive toward me was increasing, as he felt moved to bond more intensely to me: "I imagined attacking you with a two-by-four. I was going to say something about having your brains go all over the place, and then the image went down to your body, which somehow seems more awful to me, maybe because I saw my mother all bruised after my father had beaten her, and having thoughts again of you being ugly yesterday. . . . I don't want bad things for you! But maybe I can understand the reason I have these nasty thoughts, and, yea, how can I deny I have these thoughts? But that's not what I'm all about, and I get beyond the squirming and see that's not the part of me in control."
>
> (Haft, 2005, p. 1115)

> One day, the patient shared the 'vague' thought of "I'll kill you," and then suddenly remembered his father yelling "I'll kill you" to his mother, while swinging a toy hatchet. "I *think* it was a toy . . . it certainly could have killed my mother," John said hesitantly, thinking of mother dodging father the hatchet swinging out of father's hands.

> "I have a memory of . . . burying the hatchet . . . buried it to make my mother safe." In the literal-mindedness typical of this disorder, this reconstructed memory of John's expressed the hallmark of the obsessive-compulsive dynamic: distancing from (burying) one's aggression (that is, one's hatchet) in order to keep loved ones safe.
>
> (Haft, 2005, p. 1115)

The fourth sequence suggests the trajectory of therapeutic action. The analyst repeatedly interprets John's fear of contaminants (and other external hazards) as a displaced fear of his own destructive impulses and phantasies. He gradually seems to understand her: "I'm starting to get the idea of wanting to be careful to protect people from me."

We see the psychic efficacy of the interpretation in the patient's associations: a link develops, in the workings of his mind, between his own sadism and his father's aggression. He again imagines beating the analyst, for instance, and scattering her brains across the room. He now links the image of the mutilated analyst with the memory of his mother's bruised and bloodied body. He later associates from the vague thought, "I'll kill you," to a memory of his father yelling, "I'll kill you," to his mother while swinging a toy hatchet. He remembers finding the hatchet afterwards and burying it for his mother's safety.

The most salient point, from the perspective of this inquiry, is that the interpretation *does not* include the hypothesis of a retreat from an Oedipal rivalry to an anal position. Nor does it appear that such a hypothesis is needed. The interpretation given, and elaborated in the patient's associations, is consistent with the alternative hypothesis that the patient's obsessiveness defends him, not primarily against anal wishes, but against his identification with an aggressive phallic father in the Oedipal situation.

The interpretation of the patient's father identification works, to continue, against the aforementioned enactment in which the patient is figured as an unthreatening little boy. The analyst breaks from her implicit identification with Betty: She establishes that, contrary to John's transference expectations, she can perceive and survive his phallic aggression.

From Phallic-Genital to Anal Wishes/Anxieties

The hypothesis of an anal regression would suggest a diminishment of phallic-genital wishes/anxiety and a corresponding increase in anal preoccupations. The process material suggests, by contrast, an oscillation between phallic-genital and anal interests within a broadly obsessional landscape. The anal organization, which constitutes one resting place, seems part and parcel, but not uniquely determinative, of the obsessional organization.

Obsessive-Compulsive Symptoms/Behaviors

The claim of an anal regression suggests a cause-effect relationship between the shift to anality and the rise of obsessional defense. The process material suggests that the patient uses obsessional defenses to ward off sadistic-erotic impulses identified with his abusive phallic father. The defenses do not seem uniquely aimed at managing anal sadism.

Uniqueness

Contrary to expectations, there is nothing uniquely anal about John's obsessional presentation. It is possible that, in his obsessional solution, John taps earlier anal-phase experiences of toilet training and feces management. The process material does not disconfirm that classical hypothesis. Whether or not it is true, we see later precursors of the solution in his Oedipal and latency-age efforts to protect his mother against his father's abuse. Once he had identified with his father, as manifest in his pet-abuse and early adulthood treatment of women, it became imperative to protect the world against himself. He perfected an obsessional, self-emasculating defense in his relationship with Betty, on whom he still depends, yet whom he pictures himself to be defending against the world. The defensive strategy, an outcome of cumulative development, now manifests in the transference in his obsessional efforts to manage the symbols of genital aggression.

Discussion

The theory of anal regression captures something of the patient's reliance on obsessional defenses to ward of aggressive impulses. He does seem to externalize his aggression in the form of external hazards, especially contaminants, which he must then manage to protect himself and his objects. The analyst shows that, by interpreting his aggression, she helps him to move toward greater integration and a more consistent ownership of previously disclaimed wishes and impulses.

The theory is misleading, however, in this particular case, in its postulation of a unique cause-effect relation between the shift to an anal organization and the emergence of obsessional mechanisms. The obsessional mechanisms appear to be directed not at anal impulses per se (a claim which depends on the tautological equation of messy things with feces), but at impulses forged in identification with his Oedipal father and elaborated in his pet-abuse and early dating experiences.

The most useful element of the theory, then, is the link between obsessional neurosis and unmanageable hostility. I suggest that we can discard the anal regression hypothesis and retain the essential point: that obsessional defenses evolved, across the lifespan, to manage aggressive impulses.

To disconfirm the theory's regression-specific expectations is not to falsify the regression theory itself. One might argue, for instance, that the patient did regress to an anal fixation in the infantile unconscious. The anal wishes and impulses, it would be held, are too deep to manifest directly in the empirical process. They show up, one might say, in the way in which phallic impulses are expressed. The expression of phallic impulses as messy contaminants, for instance, suggests an anal hermeneutic: Semen and penis symbols are treated regressively as if they were dirty feces.

The problem with that position, as I have argued in Chapter 2, is that it creates a tautology. The analyst is left with a theory that cannot be questioned and essentially becomes its own evidence: The patient is anal because he is preoccupied with messy things; and he is preoccupied with messy things because he is anal. The tautology thwarts an open-minded analytic inquiry into the evolving, lifespan significance of messy things in the patient's internal world.

To reject the tautology is to re-open analytic inquiry into the meaning of messiness and to obtain, by extension, a more accurate and comprehensive picture of the patient's obsessional organization.

Note

1 Extracts from the case of John featured in this chapter are taken from 'On My Way Here, I Passed a Man with a Scab": Understanding a Case of Severe Obsessive-Compulsive Disorder' by Jacqueline Haft (2005). *The Psychoanalytic Quarterly* 74(4): 1101–1126, 2005. Reprinted by kind permission of the journal and Taylor & Francis, LLC.

Chapter 9

The Case of Kyle

In this chapter, I examine the case report of a restorative regression (Grossmark, 2012).[1] The case illustrates what the analyst conceptualizes as a non-defensive regression to a primary object relation (Balint, 1965, 1968). The regression, it is held, enables the patient to find his own idiosyncratic path toward a greater sense of vitality, or aliveness, in the world.

The case conceptualization rests on the theory of the primary object love (Balint, 1952, 1959, 1968). The theory suggests that 'basic fault' patients, who have suffered preverbal ruptures in maternal attunement, will experience the analyst's adult language as a self-alienating impingement. The analyst's interpretations will register, further, as so many demands and seductions: an implicit expression of the analyst's will to control the patient. His separate thoughts, feelings and intentions will feel like hard objects to be navigated. The provision of an unobtrusive relationship allows the patient, by contrast, to regress to a primary object relation, before the origin of sexual or aggressive conflict, so that he can relax and find his way, without any external pressure, to a new beginning in life.

The patient is, indeed, sensitive to the implicit power moves at play in routine analytic interpretation. He insists on a pliable, unobtrusive relationship, which does, in fact, help him to relax some and to find his way toward a new sense of his own affective presence.

The regression-specific claims, however, seem at odds with the reported process material. The patient does not seem bothered by adult language; he does not seem intolerant of the analyst's separateness per se; nor does he demonstrate a diminishment of sexual or aggressive conflict. The patient–analyst relationship does not, moreover, seem uniquely characteristic of the mother–infant bond. It seems instead that we require a full lifespan history to adequately capture the transference-countertransference. We can reject the regression hypothesis, but retain the essential insight: that the patient insists on a pliable, non-interpretive analytic relationship, not just as a defense, but as a means of growth.

The image of the patient as a needy-infant becomes a field character. The patient behaves in an imperious manner. The analyst, in turn, tempers his own frustration by picturing him as if he were a psychological baby. To temper his frustration is to lessen the guilt the analyst feels (and reports) for his underlying wish to exert control over the patient.

The needy-infant character is just one of many other characters at play in the field. It becomes a compliment, most importantly, to the totalitarian dictator of the patient's phantasy life, which, I suggest, represents the wish to humiliate and subjugate dependents.

The Primary Object

The first task is to clarify the analyst's theoretical position and the expectations it yields. Grossmark (2012) integrates strands of thought from a variety of psychoanalytic traditions. In my reading of his case, I shall focus narrowly on his use of Balint's (1968) theory of benign regression. The aim is not to give a comprehensive account of the case, or of the analyst's conceptualization, but to focus in on a modern example of restorative regression.

Balint (1968) argued that the privileged status of interpretation in psychoanalysis reflected a bias toward classical patients whose ego strength enabled them to use verbal interpretation:

> The original conflicts, as well as the defensive mechanisms and processes mobilized for coping with them, have become—and largely remain—internal events in these patients.
>
> (Balint, 1968, p. 8)

> An important precondition for internalization is a fairly good ego structure that can withstand, and contain, the tensions caused by internalization without breaking down and without resorting to a different type of defense—which may be called externalization—such as, for example, acting out, projection, confusion, denial, depersonalization.
>
> (Balint, 1968, p. 9)

> Throughout this process of conveying and reflecting, each of the two partners—patient and analyst understands reliably in the same sense what the other says. True, resistances are encountered, which may at times even be highly intense, but one can always count on a reliable and intelligent ego that is able to take in words and then allow them in influence itself.
>
> (Balint, 1968, p. 9)

The patient, in this classical model, can hear interpretations with a minimum of defensive distortion. He can do so, it is held, because he has the ego capacity to tolerate internal conflict. He is less reliant than others on defenses that twist and warp the meaning of words.

The classical patient's capacity to use interpretation, however, reflected something prior to ego strength. He was organized, Balint (1968) held, at the 'Oedipal level' of development, which, due to concurrent language acquisition, made his experience verbal. The verbal nature of his internal life rendered it subject to verbal interpretation.

Technical difficulties emerged, by contrast, with the patient unable to use verbal interpretation. The patient in question tended to hear interpretations as a 'something else.' They felt like seductions, attacks, demands, gestures of affection, reassurances etc.:

> The description just given, of our technique, presupposes that interpretations are experienced by both patient and analyst as interpretations and not as something else.
>
> (Balint, 1968, p. 9)

> The analyst may try, as hard as he can, to make his interpretations clear and unequivocal; the patient, somehow, always manages to experience them as something utterly different from that which the analyst intended them to be. At this level, explanations, arguments, improved or amended versions, if tried, prove of no avail; the analyst cannot but accept the bitter fact that his words in these areas, instead of clarifying the situation, are often misunderstood, misinterpreted, and tend to increase the confusion of tongues between his patient and himself. Words become, in fact, unreliable and unpredictable.
>
> (Balint, 1968, p. 175)

> Words—at these periods—cease to be vehicles for free association; they have become lifeless, repetitious, and stereotyped; they strike one as an old worn-out gramophone record, with the needle running endlessly in the same groove. . . . The analyst then discovers to his despair and dismay that, in these periods, there is no point whatever in going on interpreting the patient's verbal communications.
>
> (Balint, 1968, p. 175)

> The interpretation is either experienced as interference, cruelty, unwarranted demand or unfair impingement, as a hostile act, or a sign of affection, or is felt so lifeless, in fact dead, that it has no effect at all.
>
> (Balint, 1968, p. 175)

The patient and analyst became involved, through the interpretation, in a complex relational dance. The insight-value was less important than the implicit force of the comments. The force frequently registered in the sphere of power, dominance and seduction.

Balint (1968) regarded this presentation as the sign of an historical missatunement in the mother–infant dyad. The missatunement reflected a mismatch in the child's constitution and the mother's care. The child's needs might have been 'too exacting' (1968, p. 22.) The mother's response might have been, "deficient, haphazard, over-anxious, over-protective, harsh, rigid, grossly inconsistent, incorrectly timed, over-stimulating, or merely un-understanding or indifferent." The child's pain, which occurred in the preverbal years, was still felt deeply, and could be talked about, but not verbalized directly.

The patient lives, in adulthood, with the conscious feeling of living with an inner 'fault.' He yearns to be recognized and understood by an unobtrusive other. He is terrified, however, by the prospect of lowering his guard and tacitly opening himself up to be re-traumatized. He makes "a desperate demand that this time the analyst should not—in fact must not—fail him" (p. 21). The analyst, who wants to help, and perhaps to prove his own goodness, might find himself in phantasy in the role an omnipotent parent, who can protect and re-parent the patient, and who is too self-aware to fall into the feared repetition.

The analyst who presents himself as an omnipotent object, for example, in overconfident interpretation, or in an effort to demonstrate unwavering sympathy, unwittingly invites a malignant regression. The patient unconsciously elicits the analyst's phantasy and is primed by his own yearnings to reinforce it. The analyst's inevitable failure to heal the basic fault leads to new cravings and intensified demands with a deepened sense of futility.

If the analyst can be an unobtrusive presence, without too many demands or omnipotent promises, he will find that the patient is quite defended against the very care he longs for. In response to the original fault, or rupture, the patient has developed a 'shell,' in which he still lives, more-or-less adapted to reality, but restricted in his experience of life:

> This shell has a double function. It supplies the individual with various skills necessary for life, but at the same time it restricts his possibilities of experiencing either love or hatred, either joy or misery. Life will reach him only with such intensity and in such form as his shell allows.
>
> [Balint, 1959, p. 107]

The shell thus limits the experience of surrender and dependency for which the patient yearns.

Balint (1959, 1968) differentiated between 'ocnophilic' and 'philobatic' shell types. The ocnophil clings to her objects, as if they were part of her shell, intolerant of separateness, frustration and disappointment, which, though inevitable, seem to her to reconfirm the unreliability of relationships. The real aim, which cannot be achieved by clinging, is "to be held by the object and not to cling desperately to it; this being held should happen without even the need to express any wish for it" (1959, p. 34). The philobat, by contrast, lives in the illusion that "apart from his own proper equipment he needs no objects, certainly no one particular object" (p. 35). He is like a pilot safe in the skies. To him the world consists of "friendly expanses dotted more or less densely with dangerous and unpredictable objects" (p. 34). As long as he can navigate the dangers, relying entirely on himself, with plenty of open space, he can feel safe, confident and even trusting. He becomes terrified, however, when, through his own longing for contact, he finds himself involved in a relationship, unable to predict and control his object.

The analyst must adapt to the patient's characterological way of managing his objects. He lets himself be engaged, in the act of adaptation, not as an external object of desire/hate, not as a thinking/experiencing subject, but as something like a primary substance:

> The analyst's role in certain periods of new beginning resembles in many respects that of the primary substances or objects. He must be there; he must pliable to a very high degree; he must not offer too much resistance; he certainly must be indestructible, and he must allow his patient to live with him in a sort of harmonious interpenetrating mix-up.
>
> (Balint, 1968, p. 136)

> No oppressive or demanding object should be present . . . the environment should be quiet, peaceful, safe, and unobtrusive. . . . It should be there and . . . should be favorable to the subject, but . . . the subject should be in no way obliged to take notice, to acknowledge, or to be concerned about it.
>
> (Balint, 1968, p. 180)

> Only one partner may have wishes, interests, and demands on his own; without any further need for testing, it is taken for granted that the other partner, the object, or the friendly expanse, will automatically have the same wishes, interests and expectations.
>
> (Balint, 1968, p. 70)

> The guiding principle during these periods is to avoid any interference not absolutely necessary; interpretations particularly should be scrutinized most meticulously, since they are felt more often than not as unwarranted demand, attack, criticism, seduction, or stimulation; they should be given only if the analyst is certain that the patient *needs* them, for at such times *not giving them* would be felt as an unwarranted demand or stimulation.
>
> "Balint, 1968, p. 180"

To allow for such a relationship to emerge, it is essential that the analyst must be pliable. He must tolerate a high degree of acting out. He must, moreover, allow the patient to regulate the relationship, and the latent anxiety, without making unwanted interpretations, which function, in the countertransference, as an assertion of his separate mind. If he does interpret to the patient, he does so not to make the unconscious conscious, although that might happen, but rather because the patient seems to authorize it, and by the analyst's intuition, it would be felt as a demand or seduction to withhold a comment.

The result, a 'benign regression' to the level of the basic fault, manifests, in part, in the diminishment of Oedipal conflict, that is, rivalry and sexual conflict in triangular relationships (Balint, 1968, p. 15). The signs and symptoms of genital conflict, for example, hysteria, are absent (p. 146). Aggressive and destructive impulses, and the consequent persecutory anxieties and guilt feelings, which generate internal conflict, also calm down (p. 70). Balint thus asserts that, "the nature of the dynamic force operating at this level is not that of a conflict" (p. 16). The dynamic force is a preverbal yearning for the primary object.

When hatred does emerge, it is thought to reflect not a triangular situation of rivalry or competition, but, rather, a hatred of dependency, exacerbated by any disruptions. The logic is that hatred develops in reaction to the terrors of dependency on a more powerful object. The analyst's pliability, and the patient's strengthened sense of self, enable him to tolerate the situation with less resentment of their inequality (p. 71). The terror and humiliation of the dependency are reduced and, with them, the feelings of hatred.

Expectations

The theory of benign regression leaves the analyst with a set of process-oriented expectations. Listed are four expectations relevant to the notion that a regression has occurred:

1. Adult language will appear developmentally inappropriate to the patient's inner experience.
2. The patient will experience the analyst's separate thoughts, feeling and initiatives as hard objects.
3. Once the benign regression has been established, and a harmonious mix-up has emerged, the patient will experience a diminishment of sexual and aggressive conflict.
4. The interaction will, if the analyst can adapt, and if the patient can relax his defensive shell, be uniquely characteristic of a harmonious mother–infant relationship.

Questions

We can formulate these regression expectations in a set of process-oriented questions:

1. Does adult language appear developmentally inappropriate to the patient's inner experience, manifest, for instance, in his subjective sense of being misunderstood by it?
2. Does the patient feel disrupted by signs of the analyst's separate mind, manifest, for instance, in increased feelings of despair, self-alienation, noisy symptoms, or acting out?
3. Is there a diminishment of sexual and aggressive conflict, manifest, for instance, in fewer symbolic representations and/or in fewer erotic or sado-masochistic enactments?
4. Is the interaction uniquely characteristic of the posited mother–infant relationship, manifest, in positive terms, in the presence of features not equally characteristic of later object relations, and, in negative terms, in the absence of later emerging phantasies, defenses and solutions?

The Patient

The analyst, upon meeting Kyle in the initial consultation, was struck by the imagery, in his own mind, of an infant being dropped. It was an infant, further, who seemed able to communicate not primarily through words, but through action and sensory experience:

> Entering my office for the first time seven years ago, a tall, slightly chunky, and stylishly dressed blond man in his twenties with thick glasses and an intense gaze, he stood in front of the couch facing me and then seemed to let his body fall into a sitting position on the couch. I understood that he inhabited his body and being in a very particular way, and figured that his body was already telling me a story of falling, of being dropped, and that much of our work and communication was going to be in the realm of physical sensation and action; his and mine.
>
> His speech, very articulate and full of psychological insight, came at me like a pulse, an unstoppable tsunami of word-things. His words continued to come at me and into me, sometimes slamming, sometimes penetrating and sometimes caressing. Always totally physical.
>
> (Grossmark, 2012, p. 634)

The analyst's experience and portrayal of the patient implicitly suggests a link between the adult presentation and an infantile experience of being dropped. It implies that he was left with an inner chaos of sensation and affect communicable only through action and tone.

Amidst the barrage of words, the analyst pieced together a present-day picture of deep despair, procrastination and withdrawal, manifest in his studies and in his failing relationship:

> He told me that he was struggling with deep depression for which he had been in therapy since he was a teenager. He had just moved to be with his boyfriend and had ended a therapy of a few years, which had helped him with procrastination while he had been in graduate school. In New York he had consulted with a few therapists and had yet to find someone with whom he felt comfortable. He told me that he was struggling with powerful feelings of hopelessness and familiar impulses to shut himself away in his apartment and withdraw from the world, something he had done repeatedly in recent years. He and his boyfriend of seven years were fighting with increased frequency and their sex life had dwindled to almost no contact at all. His boyfriend had become very overweight, and neither seemed to be attracted to the other anymore. He was not working and was unsure what his next move would be. The boyfriend was independently wealthy and had a prosperous career, and Kyle experienced no urgency to find his own income. Kyle knew something was very wrong with him and his life.
>
> (Grossmark, 2012, pp. 634–635)

The present problems can be seen as symptomatic of an internal infancy. They raise the possibility, however, of repetitions in work-identity and intimacy (see Chapter 5), which might, in a cyclical causality, reinforce infantile precursors and complicated them in new ways.

A sense of numb non-existence seemed to pervade the patient's private experience:

> I gathered that when he would withdraw into himself, he would disappear into a timeless zone, a numb haze where he would become immersed in reading or the Internet and would exist completely out of time, forgetting to wash, eat or sleep. Hence the 'procrastination' of his graduate studies.
>
> (Grossmark, 2012, p. 635)

> He had grown up, it emerged, with the persistent thought that he did not exist. Throughout his life he felt that he was a figure in someone else's dream, and that when they would wake up, he and all the world around him would no longer exist.
>
> (Grossmark, 2012, p. 637)

The sense of non-existence was not something to which he regressed, but, at least in his subject recall during the sessions, something he had always felt and had never emerged from.

The patient described a complicated dependency on his mother, a seemingly dominant and reactive woman, whom he portrayed as micro-managing the details of his life. Behind the battle of wills there appeared a vaguely recognized wish, on his part, to let himself be managed, which he expressed in a masochistic register, but then fiercely resisted:

> At the center of his world was his mother. "She is a good person, but . . . " He described her total involvement and impingement on his life. Most recently, via almost constant phone contact, she and her current husband had chosen all his graduate school courses and guided his day-today schedule and activities, although he attended school in another state. The relationship was laced with aggression and hatred and utter dependence. "She's a severe borderline personality disorder. It's all mood swings and tantrums," he said. He described screaming fights. "When she flips, I flip." "The thing is, I love my mother, but I need time to myself. I need to make decisions, to motivate myself." When he had told her that he was in a relationship with a man, she had shown up the next day to intervene and to take him home. He resisted, but some months later he was duped into visiting home for a 'family crisis.' "They trapped me, which was OK, I guess: my life was going nowhere." He did subsequently reunite with his boyfriend.
>
> (Grossmark, 2012, p. 635)

The manifest focus is on his mother's controlling personality and volatile temperament. There is an implicit identification with her volatility: "When she flips, I flip." Behind the identification seems to be a passive wish to be 'trapped,' perhaps the masochistic expression of a wish to be held and guided, which he minimizes in his narration of the relationship. Though he felt duped into returning home, for example, it also felt okay to be trapped.

The patient's family history was further complicated by confusion, on the analyst's part, and, the analyst infers, on the patient's part, about who his 'father' was. A step-father emerges, from the swirl of potential father figures, as shifting character: He could be cool and relaxed when they smoked pot, but, when sober, became terrifying and violent:

> I tried to get a grip on the narrative of his and his family's life, but, as was to become so familiar to me with Kyle, I'd become so flooded and confused that coherence was impossible. I did gather that his biological father had left his mother before he was born, that there had been some unsuccessful attempts at reunion, that he had been brought up primarily by his mother and her second husband, whom he referred to as his 'father,' that there were two other major relationships in his mother's life. All of these men were referred to interchangeably as 'my father.' His mother was one of ten Irish American children in a large, extended, and alcoholism-dominated family. I could not sort out who were the mother's cousins and who the siblings; all were referred to as 'my cousin,' 'my uncle,' and so on, by Kyle. And to round things off nicely, some had the same names. Listening to all of this, I was imbibing the profound confusion that was the hallmark of his being.
>
> (Grossmark, 2012, p. 635)

> I found myself continually confused. At first I panicked and would ask questions in a futile attempt to gain clarity, interrupting his flow of words. Explanations did not help. I learned that I had to settle into this felt world of confusion and near-psychosis, and somehow to find a way to get comfortable, or at least survive and keep my own mind intact. About a year into the treatment his 'father' died of a sudden heart attack, and I felt like I was falling into a deep pit, desperately trying to grab onto something to help me. Who, in fact, had died? For months he became embroiled in a lawsuit; he was the only beneficiary and there was a common-law wife who legally fought him and stole all the belongings from the deceased 'father's' house. It did, eventually, become clear that the man who had died was his mother's first spouse after his biological father had disappeared from the scene. "We had a great relationship for a while," Kyle said. "We'd get high on pot together." My mind would scurry for a lifeline, a timeline. Hadn't this man been in his life when he was a young boy? They must have

> been getting high together when he was what? 11? 12? 13? 'But,' Kyle went on, "once the violence started things were never the same, and it never stopped." This father had systematically terrorized him and his mother for a number of years before finally leaving. The only relief had been getting high together. He was now inheriting some considerable amount from this man.
>
> (Grossmark, 2012, pp. 635–636)

The step-father figure seems, in Kyle's recollection, to have offered some respite from the mother, for instance, when they got high together, only to transform into a terrifying and abusive figure in his own right. He now found himself in the complicated position of being dependent (again) on this seductive-abusive character in the form of a large inheritance.

In spite of Kyle's ostensibly cool and dismissive attitude toward the many interchangeable father figures, he worked hard to stay in touch with his biological father's parents. He made it difficult, in his narration, to determine the biological father link:

> The closest and most meaningful relationship in his life seemed to be with his 'grandparents.' It took me some time to figure out that they were the parents of his biological father. Kyle made great efforts over time to visit and maintain a meaningful relationship with them.
>
> (Grossmark, 2012, p. 635)

The obscuring act here and elsewhere might indicate a need to deny the implicit father hunger.

In Kyle's latency and early adolescence, we find the development of defensive solutions, for example, sexualization, manic omnipotence, and a seeming identification with his domineering objects, which persisted, with various elaborations, into the contemporary presentation:

> He masturbated compulsively from age 7 or 8. From age 14 or so he regularly had sex in public bathrooms with men. He describes being popular in those environments, where older men would perform oral sex on him or mutually masturbate. More panic on my part, as this world of abuse unfolded, but I did register that as he described sex, I felt that we actually had a subject, almost even a focus, and my mind could almost settle into a groove. Aha: an abuse narrative. This was, of

> course, the power of sex. He, as I, in these moments, could fleetingly feel oriented in a reality, in the space of the physical/sexual. As an adult his sexuality had been a zone of compulsion, psychological grounding, and mad manic omnipotence. He told me with a sense of jaded pride: "When it comes to sex and drugs, I've done everything. Outside of heroine, I've done every drug. Outside of dead bodies and children, I've done everything sexually." Indeed, he would go to great lengths to find an experience of ever-increasing arousal: defecating in a man's mouth, watching a woman have sex with a dog, beating men on their testicles until they threw up in pain are just some of the experiences he described. "I feel like a god; I can treat a man like a toilet." "I am above the laws of reality. I can come while he throws up in pain. I am a god."
>
> (Grossmark, 2012, p. 636)

He seems to have, in part, sexualized his need for a father and, at the same time, reversed the power dynamic. He built himself up to be, and found men who colluded in his wish to be, a godlike object of desire and willful dispenser of abuse.

Beneath the sadism, erotization, and insistence on his own omnipotence was a latent depression, which he first expressed, in private, in his adolescent journals:

> He began to open his adolescent journals and we'd look at them in sessions. The sadness and constant longing to be dead. The daily onslaught of screaming fights and frequent violence. An obsessive interest in the Aztecs. They feared the sun wouldn't rise the next day, so they would make human sacrifices to the gods to be sure that the sun would indeed rise.
>
> (Grossmark, 2012, p. 637)

The entries reveal a helpless despair, in contrast to his sense of godlike omnipotence, marked by a dependency on terrifyingly powerful and demanding figures outside of his control.

Clinical Process

In the following, I shall report three clinical sequences from Grossmark's case history. The sequences consist of summarized sessions, interspersed with poignant moments from individual sessions, which the analyst has chosen to highlight. This broad-view reporting style, to its benefit, illustrates a macro-process played out over a long time period. The disadvantage is that, without the micro-process, it is more difficult to see the analyst's clinical data, and, in consequence, to identify aspects of the moment-by-moment interaction that might complicate, or call into question, features of the meta-narrative.

> *Sequence 1*
>
> He'd miss appointments and offer no explanation. He'd call in for sessions sometimes on time, sometimes late. On numerous occasions I thought he had dropped out, only to answer the phone when it rang at the time of his session and hearing him start talking; no "Hello, this is Kyle," just picking up the session from where we'd left off some time ago. I was living in a world where one is continually forgotten and where one fears that everything can be gone with no reason or warning and where there are tears in the fabric of time.
>
> He always paid for all scheduled sessions. The phone sessions became more bizarre and difficult to manage. A half hour into a session, he's mention that he was driving in the car with his mother, or had a friend sitting next to him. He'd disappear for weeks and call, and only after a while mention that he was in Thailand or Indonesia with his boyfriend. No mention of whether he might have informed me. The prize goes to the session where I heard a persistent noise while we talked, and in response to my inquiry, he mentioned, "Oh, I'm in the shower." What country was he in? I didn't feel it really mattered at that point.
>
> I tried to set some limits. More than with anything else, I was struggling with the unannounced absences. I addressed the issue and said that treatment required a more coherent structure, that he be present and at least give notice of his upcoming movements: seemingly ordinary boundary requirements. He was furious. The treatment almost ended. He was persistent and absolutely solid in his conviction. "That is your problem, not mine. This is me. I can't do this any other way," and so on. I was very affected by his rage with me. I felt deeply that I was in error to have tried to impose this structure on him, that it was my need to take back some power, some purchase on the out-of-control

> feeling that permeated the treatment. I could find no other thought in my head: He was right. This was about me, what I could or would not let myself tolerate.
>
> It's so simple. Listen to the patient and be the analyst that the patient needs you to be. Not the analyst you think you are, or ought to be. I actually found this completely liberating. Was this masochism on my part, or 'surrender' (Ghent, 1990)? Probably a bit of both, but once I allowed the experience in, and ceased trying to get him to talk about our relationship, to understand what was going on; once I allowed myself to flow with him, and "abandon any attempt at organizing the material," the treatment changed. In retrospect, I believe that his rage and insistence paradoxically provided a container for the treatment at that time, and enabled me to relax my own anxieties about his absences and dysregulation. . . . I believe that here we see Kyle protecting his own treatment and containing his analyst's fears, such that we and the treatment could thrive in his own idiom.
>
> (Grossmark, 2012, pp. 636–637)

The patient treats the sessions with a defiantly casual, but at the same time deadly serious, air. The analyst feels drawn in and then abandoned with no explanation and, it seems, a maddening sense that, in his effort to engage, he lets his needs and standards be disregarded. The invitation in sometimes takes on a seductive tone. He finds himself, for instance, in the position of a voyeur listening in on the patient's shower. But lest he indulge in the intimacy, or feel too privileged, he is shown, with an indifferent air, that at any moment a third person might turn out to be present (e.g., the mother or friend). The analyst is thus invited in, titillated, made to feel important, and then shamed for wanting more.

The analyst, in his eventual effort to set limits, evokes the patient's rage. The patient convinces him that, behind his rationalizations, he is acting out of his own need for control. The analyst is left feeling guilty for having attempted to impose his own demands.

A sadomasochistic enactment, with an exhibitionistic/voyeuristic flavor, has unfolded. The patient, in a series of sadistic-exhibitionistic moves, has dismantled the analyst's framework and drawn him into a precarious position of submission and voyeuristic intrigue. The analyst has been seduced and humiliated for his complicity and for wanting something more. The analyst has tried, out of a conscious clinical rationale, but more deeply, from a position of frustration and humiliation, to re-establish his sense of control. The display of force leaves him in a guilty-identification with the sadistic position.

It might be that the analyst identifies with a split off and projected figure from the patient's internal world. That figure would seem to represent the patient's hateful and dominant qualities, which, in turn, seem identified with the dominant mother and abusive step-father. The analyst's introduction of guilt and concern might reflect the emergence, in the repetition, of a new potentiality, a possibility unique to this field, not present in the patient's experience of himself, nor present, it seems, in his experience of his parents' minds.

The analyst manages his guilt by submitting/surrendering (a tension he leaves open) to the patient's relational style. Instead of fighting the patient, he begins to 'flow' with him. He explains his pliability, and, I infer, restores a sense of analytic integrity, through the idea that the patient, who lived in a "not-alive twilight zone," needs time to linger in an unobtrusive environment so that he might find his own way to a feeling of existence (p. 637).

The analyst's technical approach hinges on a particular view of the patient's development:

> I believe that the failures in holding and containing, along with the annihilating intrusiveness of his mother and the environment, kept from him the experiences that would have fostered an *existence*. He had no object or environmental constancy, and consequently could not trust that either he or the world would exist from one moment to the next. The treatment hinged on my being able to live in this ongoing nonexistence and know it and tolerate it, and *expect no more*. In the words of Balint: "to create an environment, a climate in which" the patient and analyst "can tolerate the regression in a mutual experience." (p. 177)

The developmental narrative is one of the basic fault. The technique is aimed, in accordance with this understanding, in minimizing demands and allowing for a benign regression.

I suggest that, whether or not the reader agrees with the analyst's conceptualization, the image of the patient as a thwarted infant, in an inconsistent mother–infant dyad, emerges in the transference-countertransference field and has an effect. The effect, in the immediate situation, is, I believe, to help the analyst manage his frustration. It is easier to tolerate in a disorganized infant what would be intolerable in a grown man. He becomes better able, in consequence, to adapt to the patient's demands, with less humiliation, since he has a clinical rationale, and so less hate and less crippling guilt.

Sequence 2

Sessions were often filled with news items from the press and political discussions. He wanted to know my points of view on a variety of political and historical questions. The theme of much of the discussions was power, cruelty and domination. He wanted to know about my family background, my family history. He became very involved with the Holocaust and read voluminously. I would speak openly and honestly to him. I left the question of the analyst's self-revelation many miles behind. I understood that he needed someone to partner with, to think with, to know, and be known by, in a non-impinging manner, someone with whom he could "dream himself into existence" in the words of Ogden (2009, p. 15). As Winnicott suggested, often these sessions did not appear to be anything like analysis or therapy. The crises of the Middle East, the troubles of Northern Ireland, the role of the Ukranians in World War II, the Chavez regime in Venezuela, and so on. On occasion he'd email me long essays that he'd written, or articles that he had found on the web, and he'd want to engage me in discussion about them. I would be with him in these discussions and only engage with the personal relevance to him on the rare occasions when he would offer it. For instance, he commented when talking about imperialism, that he understood now that his mind had been 'colonized' by his mother's madness.

Generally, I was unobtrusive while being totally and intimately engaged. I'd silently make connections to myself tracking my reverie and my thought about his psychic process, while engaging in these discussions with sincerity and real interest. My strong feeling in these times is opposite of what one hears most frequently, across psychoanalytic approaches: it is OK for these kinds of extra-therapy interactions or enactments to occur, as long as they are talked about or analyzed after. My feeling was that it was of utmost importance that I enter these interactions as me, unadorned; and it was equally important, that

> they were not talked about after, unless he brought in the kind of connection such as the one I mentioned about his being colonized.
>
> (Grossmark, 2012, p. 638)

The rupture of the previous sequence led the analyst to relinquish his former expectations and realign around the patient's agenda. The atmosphere seems to calm down. The patient seems to explore his own feelings of power, cruelty and domination through the intellectual discussion of genocide and totalitarianism on the world stage. He can link his interest in world oppression to his own feeling of being colonized by his mother. The analyst, however, is forbidden to make such links—not because they are inapt, or because the insight is intolerable—but because, if they come from the analyst's mind, at a time when the analyst deems fit, and not when the patient has authorized it, they are felt as a disruption.

The guiding imagery, as mentioned above, is that of the patient-as-infant. The use of intellectualization, however, to manage inner tensions, reflects the influence of later cognitive achievement, manifesting for the first-time in his adolescent diary entries about the Aztecs. Anna Freud's (1936) comments on the adolescent use of intellectualization are apt. She points out the adolescent's capacity for deep insight alongside his tendency to enact the very problems with which he preoccupies himself in the sphere of abstract ideas:

> When the prepubertal period begins, a tendency for the concrete interests of the latency period to give place to abstractions becomes more and more marked. In particular, adolescents of the type which Bernfeld describes as characterized by 'prolonged puberty' have an insatiable desire to think about abstract subjects, to turn them over in their minds, and to talk about them. Many of the friendships of youth are based on and maintained by this desire to meditate upon and discuss such subjects together. The range of these abstract interest and of the problems which these young people try to solve is very wide. They will argue the case for free love or marriage and family life, a free-lance existence or the adoption of a profession, roving or settling down, or discuss philosophical problems such as religion or free thought, or different political theories, such as revolution versus submission to authority, or friendship itself in all its forms. If, as sometimes happens in analysis, we receive a faithful report of the conversations of young

> people or if—as has been done by many of those who make a study of puberty—we examine the diaries and jottings of adolescents, we are not only amazed at the wide and unfettered sweep of their thought but impressed by the degree of empathy and understanding manifested, by their apparent superiority to more mature thinkers, and sometimes even by the wisdom which they display in their handling of the most difficult problems.
>
> (Freud, 1936, pp. 159–160)

> We are surprised to discover that this fine intellectual performance makes little or no difference to his actual behavior. His empathy into the mental processes of other people does not prevent him from displaying the most outrageous lack of consideration towards those nearest to him. His lofty view of love and of the obligations of a lover does not mitigate the callousness of which he is repeatedly guilty in his various love affairs. The fact that his understanding of and interest in the structure of society often far exceeds those of later years does not assist him in the least to find his true place in social life, nor does the many-sidedness of his interest deter him from concentrating upon a single point—his preoccupation with his own personality.
>
> (Freud, 1936, p. 160)

The inconsistency, which Anna Freud captures, is evident in the contrast between the patient's interest in totalitarianism, and his implicit effort at intellectual mastery, and simultaneous enactment of a sadomasochistic dynamic in the analysis. In the enactment, he becomes the kind of tyrant who intrigues and terrifies him. The latent anxiety, one can infer, with some support from the first sequence, is that, if he relaxes his guard, and gives full play to his dependency needs, then the tables will turn, and he will find himself in the analyst's power.

It is important to highlight the observation, in the first passage above, that many friendships of youth are based on the desire to discuss and meditate on such subjects together. It is not just a way of managing internal conflict, then, but also a way of being with others. Here we find a complication of the analyst's role in the enactment. The patient asks him about his family background and his social and political views on genocide, totalitarianism etc. The analyst grows to speak openly and honestly, leaving behind the "question of the analyst's self-revelation." He becomes,

I suggest, a complex object: at once a resting tyrant, a submissive voyeur, an unobtrusive parent, and now, in addition, a flawed and vulnerable peer, a friend with whom to share in the intimacy of ideas.

The emergence of a troubled-peer signals and develops a new opening the analytic field. The analyst-as-mother was not allowed to impose his separate thoughts. The analyst as analyst-as-mother/troubled-peer has more leeway to express his mind; in fact, it is invited. The patient, in this limited intimacy, which depends on a phantasy of equality, and a denial of the analytic asymmetry, can luxuriate in the discovery of a partner in thought.

The relationship has begun to depart, in certain important ways, from what Balint might lead one to expect of a harmonious mother–infant mix-up in the transference. An adult language—one of intellectual inquiry and dialogue—has, instead of being felt as dead or inapt, become an immediate and lively vehicle for the expression of pain, terror and hatred. The discussion topics, which represent themes of dominance and submission, suggest further that, while the analyst has become more pliable, the patient's conflicts have not diminished. Rather, the patient, who longs unconsciously for a reliable other, becomes terrified of the analyst's power. He tries to ward off his dread by reversing the power dynamic in his effort to seduce and humiliate the analyst. He thus enacts his internal conflict in the analytic relationship and, at the same time, represents it in his speech.

The analyst, moreover, is not denied the right to have separate interests but, on the contrary, is invited to share his history and express his own views, with one caveat: He cannot make analytic interpretations. He is forbidden to interpret, I suggest, not because Kyle rejects the imposition of a separate mind, which, in fact, he seems to enjoy, if it is that of a vulnerable peer, but rather because interpretations remind Kyle of the analytic asymmetry. It is authority, not intersubjectivity per se, that the patient seems unable to tolerate.

Sequence 3

As with other patient's like him, he would show rather than tell. He had liposuction surgery. He came to my office while still healing, peeled off his shirt to show me his torso, which had four small holes in [it], out of which oozed the last drops of the fat that had largely been removed. I stayed in the idiom of the moment. We talked about the liposuction treatment, the physical feeling of discomfort and his

> wishes for a leaner body, his appreciation of the doctor, who helped him feel better without questioning his motives—he had not been that overweight. I held my thoughts about his showing me the embodiment of the damaged container of his mind, the ruptures in his psychic skin and in his reality, and his appreciation for me, that I was now meeting him where he needed to be met. In the language of Bion, we witnessed the introduction into the treatment of beta elements, "something more basic, more concrete and physical than what we generally mean by feelings" (Lombardi, 2007, p. 388). As Lomdardi (2007) suggests, this process can only emerge within and through the actual physical bodies of the patient and the analyst. These elements, emerging via Kyle's body in the consulting room, were transformed, within my reverie and in the process of talking with him in his idiom, into the beginnings of alpha elements of more coherence experience.
>
> (Grossmark, 2012, p. 639)

The meeting of minds in the past sequence seemed to depend on the patient's denial of asymmetry. The analyst made a reasoned and theoretically valid choice to join with the patient in minimizing tokens of his authority (interpretations, frame issues). The latent dependency needs and terror of authority played out in intellectual discussions of history and politics. The parent/peer hybrid was an emergent field product uniquely usable to the patient.

The sensation of joining, or fitting in together, did not, however, mitigate internal conflict. Nor did it dissipate the force of the enactment. In the third clinical sequence, the patient shows that he feels joined to the analyst *in* reenacting his pattern of seduction and dominance. He strips off his shirt with almost no warning, no curiosity about the meaning, and no apparent interest in how he might be experienced, to reveal a perversely intimate display: a punctured torso oozing with fat. The patient has once again stunned the analyst into the position of a submissive voyeur, who is repulsed and yet helplessly enthralled, and who, like the men in the dungeons, is ready to receive the basest of his substances.

The patient voices appreciation for the doctor who helped him without inquiring into his motives. Whatever gratitude he might feel for the analyst, who similarly helps without interpreting, there is an implicit warning: His reasons and motives are not to be questioned. The object of gratitude is still a dangerous one who might turn on him at any moment.

The analyst seems to feel a certain judgment channeled into, or mixed in with, his curiosity. The patient, he comments, "had not been that overweight." The implication is that it was the gratuitous operation. The analyst then shifts to consider the enactment as a communication: Perhaps the patient needed a physical medium to convey the "damaged container of his mind." The imagery lends itself to a Bionian stance of non-interpretive containment, which, in this case, reinforces the prior Balintian dictum to fit in without interpreting. But he also withholds his interpretation, I suggest, because to analyze the patient's motives would feel, in light of his actual criticism, and sense of being invaded, like a rejection and, perhaps, a counter-attack in defiance of the patient's provocative intrusion. He chooses, instead of an interpretive attack, the position of masochistic voyeur.

If we consider the patient's sensitivity, furthermore, it seems plausible that he does, in fact, perceive the analyst's latent skepticism. The pressured feeling of triumph, and the insistence on not being questioned, might signal the fact that he does, in fact, feel challenged. The analyst's effort to adapt, by implication, which results in an unspeakable criticism, might, apart from his intentions, stimulate the behavior to which he must then submit.

Levenson observed, as I have mentioned, that the formal of an analytic session tends to replicate its content (see Chapter 4). Here the analyst's theoretical stance, which enables him to surrender to the patient, becomes part and parcel of the sado-masochistic enactment. In other words, the pathway of repetition is also the pathway of growth and change.

Adult Language

The patient, as Balint (1968) would lead us to expect, experiences the analyst's effort to establish a frame and to make interpretations as an unwelcome expression of his own needs and interests. This fact has little to do, however, with the inaptitude of adult language. The patient is content to express himself in adult language (e.g., the language of social-political inquiry) as long as he is the one to set the topics and to initiate any interpretations that link the material to his personal history or present internal struggles. The issue is not adult language, per se, but authority. He is at pains to mitigate his unconscious terror of being possessed and controlled by the analyst.

A Separate Mind

The basic-fault patient, in Balint's (1968) conceptualization, cannot tolerate the impingement of a separate mind. The intolerance is supposed to manifest in an aversion, perhaps masked by lifeless compliance, to the analyst's separate wishes, interests and initiatives. We do indeed find, as mentioned above, a specific aversion to signifiers of analytic authority: the asymmetrical frame and analyst-initiated interpretation. The patient does not, however, seem averse to the analyst's (separate) background and socio-political views. He does not react to the latter tokens of separateness, that is, with the same rage he directs toward interpretations and frame issues, nor with dead compliance, nor with efforts to make it seem as if he and the analyst have similar histories and socio-political ideals. The difference seems to be that, while the former represent analytic authority, and thus activate the terrors of submission, the latter, which are offered in the spirit of egalitarianism, evoke a fallible, less authoritarian and therefore more tolerable object. As with language, then, the patient is not intolerant of separateness per se, but of authority.

Sexual and Aggressive Conflict

The theory of the basic fault suggests that, in a benign regression, erotic and destructive impulses (the driving forces of later Oedipal conflict) diminish in force. The clinical material suggests, however, that, even in the second and third sequences, when the regression is thought to be established, erotic and destructive impulses—and the anxieties they evoke—retain their intensity. The patient repeatedly seduces the analyst into the position of a masochistic voyeur vis-à-vis an exhibitionistic sadist. The analyst, lest he become a tyrant, is forced to surrender control to his master-patient. The erotic-sadomasochistic repetition is, in itself, the vehicle for a new object experience. It does die down, in other words, but rather facilitates the meeting of minds.

Uniqueness

The benign regression is thought to revive an object relationship uniquely characteristic of the mother–infant dyad. It is indeed possible to reconstruct, simply on the basis of the patient's sensitivity to authority and his related fear of dependency, a mismatch of needs and early maternal provision. Such a reconstruction would be consistent with the mother's apparently domineering manner. The problem is that—if we follow the patient's experience—she has always been overly controlling. The patient's experience of her as such does not seem unique to his (reconstructed) infancy.

The above enactment seems, in addition, to reflect influences beyond the child–mother relationship. The pleasure in abusing submissive men, for example, suggest an identification with the abusive step-father and, in adolescence and young adulthood, the transformation from passive to active in the constitution of a negative identity: the self as a godly seducer and punisher of men. The performance of this negative identity instigates his intellectual effort, with an apparent adolescent onset, to master the tensions of submission and dominance in the political sphere.

The sadomasochistic enactment, then, shows the cumulative influences of every major life phase. It is not a revival of the primary mother–infant bond, but a re-iteration with novel qualities.

Discussion

The theory of the basic fault captures the patient's tendency to hear the analyst's interpretations as something else. He tends to hear them as displays of authority and a will to power. The analyst finds, following Balint's technical recommendations, that, by being pliable and unobtrusive, he can enable the patient to find his own path to a sense of vitality in relation to others.

The theory breaks down, however, in its specific claims about the features of a benign regression. We find disconfirmed a set of regression-specific expectations about the inaptitude of language, the intolerance of intersubjectivity, the weakening of sexual and destructive impulses (and the attendant diminishment of internal conflict) and the uniqueness of the mother–infant dynamic.

It seems, then, that the most useful aspects of Balint's theory are those which have little to do with regression per se. I suggest that can discard the regression hypotheses and still retain the essential point: that for some patients, like Kyle, who feel that they do not exist and are terrified of dependency, there might be periods of time when, contrary to the traditional hypothesis that interpretations enable growth, the provision of a pliable, non-interpretive atmosphere seems most facilitative.

To disconfirm Balint's regression-specific expectations is not to falsify his regression theory. A proponent of the theory might assert, for example, that there is indeed a preverbal self—the unmodified residue of actual infantile experience—in the patient's deep unconscious. It is generally assumed, in that kind of assertion, that the deep infantile self cannot be directly observed. It only manifests itself indirectly through the layers of later material. The empirical session data, which attests to later developmental influences, merely reflect these more superficial accretions. To the extent that they are present, the regression is limited, but the basic theory untouched.

The problem with that position, as discussed in Chapter 2, is that it leaves the analyst in a tautology. He is left with a theory that cannot be questioned and in effect becomes its own evidence, for example, in reconstructions of the patient's infancy. It might serve to organize the analyst's experience, and so to allay anxiety, but risks a genetic fallacy with an implicit morality of maturity.

The needy and thwarted infant in the analyst's mind might, by contrast, be considered an emergent character in the here-and-now field. It emerges in the first sequence in the aftermath of the analyst's guilt-ridden effort at self-assertion. It helps, I suggest, to temper his frustration and so lessen his guilt. It also seems to restore a temporarily threatened sense of analytic integrity: There is now a formal rational for submitting/surrendering and an implicit sense of direction in the work.

The analyst's needy-infant character seems a counterpart to the patient's totalitarian dictator. The complimentary characters reflect both sides of the terror of dependency in the room. The one represents helpless need and vulnerability; the other a will to humiliate and make subservient. The patient establishes himself in the latter position. He seems unconsciously to perceive, however, as manifest in his symptoms, that his neediness renders him vulnerable to a reversal.

A series of novel field elements render the new iteration different from a literal mother–infant dyad. We find, on the patient's side, the use of intellectualization and the seeming creation of a flawed peer-role, or phantasy, which, I suggest, helps him modulate his fear of the analyst. On the analyst's side, we find a pliability and a capacity for guilt that make him a new kind of tyrant. The novel aspects of the repetition signal an opening for psychic change: toward a capacity for dependency on a flawed other and a potential, at present realized in the analyst, for concern.

Note

1 Extracts from this case report are taken from the journal article 'The Unobtrusive Relational Analyst', Robert Grossmark (2012). *Psychoanalytic Dialogues* 22: 629–646. Reprinted by permission of the journal and Taylor & Francis, LLC.

Chapter 10

The Case of Travis

In the past two chapters, I explored recent accounts of a defensive and restorative regression, respectively. In each case, the term *regression* facilitated an inquiry into early development. The inquiry led, in turn, to plausible hypotheses about each patient in his earliest years. Little was written about how later growth had absorbed and modified early trends. It was as if later life served only to perpetuate what had already been laid down. We were left with plausible and organizing, but relatively infantocentric, analytic portraits.

The critique of regression does not aim to dispel the character of the patient-as-child. It simply highlights the character as such—as a field product, one with history, but not a pristine relic. It opens an inquiry into the function of the character in the immediate field.

In the following I present an irreversible lifespan approach in my own analytic work.[1] Travis, a 28-year-old singer-songwriter, sought analysis to address intrusive jealous phantasies. He worried in seemingly every waking moment that his lovers, of whom there were several, would cheat on him with more masculine and more successful artists. The phantasies emerged not *directly* from childhood—not from unmodified unconscious infantile wishes and anxieties—but *indirectly* through a lifespan of deferred action.

I shall first present the patient and give a brief developmental history. I then offer process notes from three sequential analytic sessions. I suggest, in my conceptualization, how a regression theorist might interpret the material. I then propose an alternative, and, I argue, more accurate reading in which Travis does not *regress*, but *progresses* into the present. In doing so, he brings old patterns into a new phase of developmental tasks and anxieties.

Travis

Travis was a short, attractive man with disheveled hair and a certain boyish shyness. He dressed in thread-bare tee-shirts with tight black jeans and worn-out tennis shoes. He walked quickly, hunched forward with a glazed stare, as if had had too much coffee and was too preoccupied to rest. In his satchel he always carried one or two classic novels and a leather-bound journal. I tended to find him reading in the waiting room.

He first sought weekly psychotherapy after a breakup because he did not trust—yet could not shake—his jealous fantasies. He believed, without clear reason, that his ex-girlfriend of four years had cheated on him. In early sessions, he went over and over times when she had felt distant, arrived a few minutes late, or laughed with another man at a party. He would then debate himself. She was, he insisted, a patient and kind-hearted friend. She wore bright cheerful colors. It wasn't in her heart to betray him. He mistrusted her one minute and recused himself the next. Nightly interrogations had, over the years, worn down her patience. She left him, but stayed in touch, insisting he find help.

The breakup was the latest in a string of similar endings. He emphasized having contemplated therapy since adolescence. He had steeped himself in self-help literature on borderline personality disorder and finally sought therapy at the urging of one text—*The Angry Heart* (Santoro, 1997). It so happened that his father was also an avid self-help reader. Travis said he needed my help in seeing through his distortions to external reality.

To this picture, he added with no sense of irony that he had cheated on nearly all of his partners. He appealed to their supposed actions: "If she's out doing whatever, why shouldn't I?" "You expect everyone to cheat," I said. "Doesn't everyone?" He asked in sincerity.

After four years of weekly and sometimes twice-weekly therapy, Travis moved into four-times-per-week analysis on the couch. At present, he has been in analysis for four additional years.

Travis was the first of two children born to teenage parents who divorced when he was three. For two years after the divorce, Travis and his little sister lived with their mother. He does not remember this time. When he was five, his father won custody of them both. For years afterwards, his father rehearsed the minute details of the judge's ruling. Still Travis cannot explain it. One day afterwards his mother pulled up at his father's house apparently on the run for writing bad checks. It was unclear what she was involved in. She was an evil woman, his father often said, one who didn't really love her son.

Travis remembers her in less dramatic terms. In his earliest memory, he watches cartoons on her couch. She folds laundry in the next room. He feels mildly bored. In latency memories, she and his grandfather ask cautiously if he feels safe at his father's house. He says yes. Secretly, he wished he could move in with them to escape his father's temper. Once a bruised arm led his mother to call child services. At his father's instruction, Travis lied to the caseworker: He tripped; his father did not throw him into the table.

Now and then, his mother would take him to a fair or the local water park. His father was suspicious of her motives. Travis often returned home to find him brooding at the kitchen table. "So what did she say?" His father would ask. "Nothing," Travis would reply. "What's that on your mouth?" "What?" "That blue crap?" "Cotton candy." "Then say so." "I did." "So, it's all fun with Mom. Not as much fun with Dad, is it?" "I dunno." "Don't lie." "I'm not." "Uh-huh. Just remember who loves you." "I know." "Do you know?"

Of the latency years, Travis recalls his father's aggressive efforts to toughen him up. One day, around age ten, his father oversaw him playing a baseball video game in the family room. Travis was winning. His father scoffed at son's delight and picked up a controller. He insisted, against his son's protest, they play each other. He struck out one of his son's players after the next. "What the hell are you doing?" He demanded to know. "Get it together." Travis lost badly. His father made him play again. "You're not leaving like that. Stop being a pussy." Finally, Travis threw the remote and ran upstairs in tears.

Travis grew into an awkward and unpopular teenager. He remembers lingering in the halls. He tracked one group of three or four boys, but never felt accepted. Somehow, he discovered a melancholy subgenre of Indie Rock. He later brought me some favorite lyrics. The singer in one song wakes up in a field after a drug binge. He walks down to a train-yard and catches a boxcar to a far-away town where he gets drunk watching the locals.

Soon Travis began to imagine himself in the mold of his favorite singer-songwriters. He learned the guitar and wrote songs in secret. He read interview after interview with his heroes and tried to adopt their attitudes. He imagined giving his own interviews. Somewhere in the crowd he would find a quiet, edgy girl who understood his loneliness.

He worried, meanwhile, about his burgeoning physique. He grew calves like boulders, almost too big for his jeans, and swelling pectorals. He looked like a varsity athlete—and hated himself for it. It was antithetical to the slender, ascetic image he found in his idols. He envied the way their clothes hung on their bodies. The wish to be slender seemed part of deeper wish to reject his masculinity. He felt—and wanted to be seen as—'feminine.' By this, he meant vulnerable, perceptive and emotionally complex. In his lyrics, he often portrayed a teenage girl, lost, dejected, searching, in need of guidance.

One day, his father found his notepad. He read the lyrics in a whiny sing-song voice. Travis' sister smirked in the background. Having refused to see her mother, she had apparently become their father's favorite. "So you think you have it bad, huh?" His father teased. He crumpled the page and threw it aside. "How about you stop bitching and do your homework." "He was right." Travis later told me. "I was just a whiny little brat."

In junior year, an attractive and popular girl took an interest in him. They dated briefly until Travis discovered that she had cheated on him with a friend. When he first confronted her, she lied. Later she admitted the truth. He was enraged—not just by the act itself, but by her effort to make him feel crazy. It crushed him to see she did not care how tenuous he already felt in his reality-testing. She was ready, on the slightest whim, to exploit his vulnerability for her own advantage. In the aftermath, he recalled a certain intimation in his father's tone toward his mother. He 'realized' his father, who had never said so directly, had spoken out of a similar hurt place. It meant his mother had cheated. The present betrayal now registered as a confirmation that women could not be trusted.

Travis soon dropped out of school, on his father's advice, to take a local factory job. In private, he kept writing and scheming to pursue music—a dream which obsessed him, but which he now also considered invalid, an expression of childish vanity and self-indulgence. At twenty, he quit his job and moved an hour away to the city to make it happen. He found flexible work in a coffee shop and went on Craig's List to find band mates.

I met him eight years later. It hadn't gone well. To his credit he had found bands. But in spite of his talent, which many recognized, he never lasted long in any group. In one emblematic scenario, he and two acquaintances rented practice space in a former psych ward. A half-empty building on a boarded-up campus, it had the perfect haunted atmosphere. Travis arrived with a strict practice agenda. After thirty minutes, the two others set down their instruments and began searching YouTube for another group's song. Travis smoked impatiently. Then he snapped at them to hurry up. They blew him off. A few repeat experiences led the group to disband. For the rest of the year, Travis commuted two hours to practice alone in the rented room. "Other people want to hang out and dick around. No one takes it seriously," he told me. "I end up looking like the asshole."

Travis often baited me to join his father in shaming him. He complained one day of a customer, a chatty regular at the coffee shop, who criticized him for his lackluster attitude. He associated to sleepless nights in his stuffy apartment. It was hot, and he had asthma, but could not afford an air conditioner and, without insurance, had no asthma inhaler. The needed inhaler—which he did not try hard to get—seemed a metaphor for his situation. He felt deprived of resources and, at the same time, unworthy of pursuing them. He was, he said, a mediocre talent. Others praised him out of pity. His real job was to flatter customers for petty cash. If he didn't do it, he could get fired. It was entitled, said the next day, to want for anything more. He should give up on his artistic ambitions. They were the vain imaginings of a self-indulgent child. "What does he want?" I asked. "Who cares?" He said. "I do," I said. "I think I should just poison the brat."

As it happened, many attractive women sought him out. He typically rejected them for their generic aesthetic tastes. He rejected one woman, for instance, whom he described as beautiful and kind, because she listened to contemporary pop music in her car. "Should I force it?" he asked me. "Can I? She's a nice person, but, I mean, come on!" He held out for muse-like figures who inspired him—a dancer, film-maker, a costume designer, a poet, a comedian. He could fall, somewhat easily it seemed to me, although to him it often felt difficult and hard-won, into a sense of intimacy and deep sharing. "I really like what she does," he said, after one date's dance performance. "It's not like [a particular ex's] dancing. That was very classical. This I could relate to. I think we could have something. I was really surprised. I could see us playing off each other."

But he could not imagine an inspired woman choosing a loser like him. He might be able to charm her, to intrigue momentarily her with his pain, but she would soon get bored. He tended to read even compliments as manipulations intended to placate him for a time. After a month or so he would, for instance, play his date a song or show her a performance on YouTube. "You're amazing," one said. The next day he had trouble speaking. He ranted about his customers, got confused and lost himself in tangents. Then he folded his arms and lay in silence. "What do you think she meant?" he said at last. " 'Amazing.' She was being nice. But she didn't ask me to send her the single. And besides, it's like what, 'Now you like me? Like you didn't like me before the song?' "

Over time, he and I learned that his jealous phantasies were strongest when he felt neglected. Even a slight lapse in attention meant, to him, that his partner wanted someone else. The other man was, in his mind, a singer-songwriter who fit better in his clothes. He would first denigrate his rivals and only with reluctance admit his feelings of envy. "Can you believe he has a man-bun?" He said of one coffee shop co-worker—a more active musician—who, at least in his fantasy life, was the object of his partner's desire. "But he dresses well . . . in a certain way. He's moving to LA with his band. Even him."

Travis resented his own jealousy. To master the implicit neediness, he dated a polyamorous woman.[2] One day she came late to his apartment. She said her parents had delayed her. She offhandedly mentioned her bus route and a last-minute delay in a Seven Eleven. The route made no sense. The store was off a different bus line: the line to her other boyfriend's place. He was also a singer-songwriter. At the time he was doing more performing. Travis was cold, but, unlike usual, fought back the impulse to call out her 'lie.'

The next day, he had a session. "You think I'm an idiot," he said. "What gives you that idea?" I said. "So she lied about coming from his place," he said. "She doesn't trust me yet. Okay. But I really like her. And I think she likes me." "And I think you're fooling yourself?" "Aren't I fooling myself?" He invited me to call him out and, in the same moment, left it open for me to surprise him. I might see something desirable in him.

The polyamorous woman left him a few weeks later. She told him he made her too anxious. He let himself believe that her anxiety derived primarily from her academic work. It seemed more realistic that, as so often happened, he had worn out her patience through an insidious reassurance-seeking by which he implied she was a naïve and fickle whore. As usual, he had secretly been seeing other women on the side. He said he wanted to stop dating and focus on music, but he lost himself almost immediately in his new partners. The sessions below were, to my mind, more or less typical of the process at this point.

The Analytic Process

First Session

Travis: Last night, I just killed it with music. I was going into the album, making these surgical corrections. I realized how much I've taught myself. My confidence was really up. The most important thing is just to spend time doing it.

[Brief pause.]

Travis: Alyssa decided that she doesn't have time for a boyfriend. We agreed to keep it casual. It was like . . . fine, you know, not a big deal. I'm seeing other people too.

[Brief pause.]

Travis: When that kind of thing happens it does make me wonder, though, like, was I not charming enough? Will I ever meet someone I like who *is* ready for a relationship? Jenna is ready, but I don't know her well enough. She comes over drunk and doesn't open up. Maria has Lindsey's smile, but seems really busy. She also has a calm polite dog, so that's a plus. Unlike Sayre's dog, which is like . . . a frantic moth.

[Brief pause.]

Travis: I want a girlfriend, but nothing is working out, so I'm not thinking about it too much.

[Brief pause.]

Travis: I just had a horrible memory. It was when Skyler and I were dating. Her ex-boyfriend's father had just died. She told me, and I thought . . . good. She had lied for so long about having friends she'd slept with. Then it would come out casually. "Oh yea, I did sleep with him." And there was something off, something so secretive about her. She always seemed to be going behind my back.

[Brief pause.]

Travis: How could I be so cut off? [Self-condemning tone]
Greg: What do you think?

Travis: He must represent someone who I feel has everything and so when something bad happens to him I feel glad about it. I think, "Well, good. What, this kid doesn't deserve to have anything bad happen to him?" Skyler will probably like to me and sleep with him again to make him feel good. She cheated on me with him! Then again, I say that but we weren't together. It shows how detached from reality I can get.

[Brief pause.]

Travis: I feel I'm living out a different reality with different people. Skyler and I were hanging out a lot, and I would tell her I wasn't dating other people. If she slept with someone else, I would react to her as if she had cheated on me. Even though *I* was seeing other people. But I wasn't pretending. I really felt that way. I would forget I was seeing other people. I don't think you or anyone else understands. I would truly forget.

Greg: I do believe you would forget in the moment. But even when I reminded you, you dismissed it. You didn't think it mattered, because, in your mind, it was a justified reaction. At first you wanted to trust her, and I believe you intended to commit to her, but after just a few weeks you started to suspect her of cheating on you. You began reading into her behavior to prove she had cheated. Then you started cheating. You would say, "Hey, I'm trying to commit to her, but she's out doing whatever she wants. So why shouldn't I?" But the problem is—in retrospect—you never really had any evidence she was cheating. It was all an assumption.

Travis: Yea . . . but you make it sound like I'm some sort of deliberate mastermind. I think I'm the only one who gets how lost I got in that reality.

Greg: I'm not saying it was your conscious intention. It was an unconscious pattern.

Travis: Oh. Yea, Okay. [Chuckles.] Well, now I can accept that Jenna and I are seeing separate people instead of getting lost in the story.

[Long pause. He seems calm, relaxed. I get the feeling he wants me to prompt him.]

Greg: What did you mean when you said that that guy has everything?

Travis: He's handsome, likable. He has Skyler on a string. I think he's doing well in his career. He's in entertainment. I think he just moved to LA. He's capable of a casual relationship. It's like, "Oh, two people actually just like each other. They're going to have sex without a commitment!"

Greg: It's validating.

Travis: It shows interest, acceptance, a genuine friendship, being enamored. Everyone has someone in their head who represents the fun attractive person who doesn't need to devote themselves to them to get attention. Then I would think the fun attractive person broke the rules, did something seedy.

Greg: Somehow it tends to be an artist or a performer.

Travis: I just picture them in the lifestyle. Tattoos, hipper clothes. Less serious. A more relaxed guy. Not me—a polite dork. All the other kids say, "Let's go play with fireworks." And I say, "No, I don't think we should." I'm lame, jealous, clean-cut, square. I'm the loser.

Discussion

Travis first asserts his newfound confidence in his music practice. We have spent many prior sessions exploring his fear that to invest in his creative work is, in essence, to indulge in an 'arrogant' self-image—the image of himself as a rock star—that he should suppress. He worries that if he indulges himself, he will ultimately discover that he is just mediocre. I hear his assertion, in context, as an appeal to his progress in overcoming his pessimism.

In asserting his progress, he attempts to bolster himself against what now troubles him: the rejection. At first, he minimizes it. But the attempted denial gives way to real concerns. He wonders when he will meet a woman who wants to date him. He briefly recounts the recent women who haven't worked out. He says dubiously that he isn't thinking much about it. He seems at pains to give any weight to the subject that is on his mind.

He associates to a troubling memory in which his ex-girlfriend Skyler, tells him that her ex-boyfriend lost his father. Travis is troubled by his thought, 'good.' He then tries to cast doubt on Skyler's fidelity. He seems to wait for me to confirm her bad character. I say nothing. He then turns back on himself. He asks in a self-condemning tone how he could be so 'cut-off' as to feel glad when her ex lost his father. I believe he has taken my silence as judgment and is now voicing what he considers to be my view of him.

I ask him how he understands it. By this question, I hope to bring his projected self-criticism into the dialogue. I think that, if he explains himself, I will have greater opportunity to explore the self-censorship he feels vis-à-vis his envious and hateful thoughts. It might eventually become possible to challenge the bond he establishes between us in which we seemingly both agree that is cut-off from the empathy he should feel.

He answers that the ex-boyfriend must represent someone he would envy and therefore want to see hurt. His reply more-or-less parallels prior interpretations I have made. It begs the question of what he was looking for in asking me to restate a now familiar comment. Perhaps he wanted me to punish him by repeating a lesson to a bad pupil.

But he cannot fully use the interpretation. He cannot use it because it implies that he should work through an unnecessary envy. He believes, on the contrary, that his envy is warranted. To justify his envy, he points out that Skyler *did* cheat on him with this ex-boyfriend. He then recalls that she slept with her ex *after* she and Travis broke up. He is thrown back on himself. He recognizes the discrepancy between his feeling of betrayal and the reality that, since they had broken up, he no longer had any claim on her attention.

He goes on to insist on his altered sense of reality. He recalls that he would profess—falsely—to be monogamously committed to Skyler. He would then accuse her of cheating on him even though he was, in truth, cheating on her. He wants me to understand that he wasn't 'pretending' to be monogamously committed. It is important for me to believe that, in the moment, he sincerely forgot that he was seeing other women.

I sense that he is overstating his forgetfulness in an effort to evade his self-criticism. I point out that even when I remind him of his own cheating, he discounts its relevance. I suggest an alternative narrative that, I think, better accounts for his momentary denial. In my alternative story, he is monogamous in intention. He assumes, however, that she will betray him. So, he lets himself stray. He then blames her, in essence, for not sharing his *intention*. In emphasizing his intention, he effectively denies the fact, which momentarily seems irrelevant to him, that he has acted in a contradictory manner. The problem, which I point out, is that he merely assumes her infidelity. The assumption reflects his low self-confidence and a priori mistrust. It hardly counts as proof.

My interpretation implicitly asks him to take greater responsibility for his conduct. I portray him as an agent who initiates, makes assumptions and reacts defensively. He rejects the portrayal. ("You make it sound like I'm some sort of deliberate mastermind.") He insists that I do not understand how lost he gets in his other reality.

At this point, I believe we have fallen into an interpersonal enactment of his self-criticism. I implicitly ask him to take greater responsibility. He insists, in something like an insanity defense, that he got lost in an alternate reality and so should be judged less severely. I imagine that he feels judged severely by me in part because he severely judges himself—or would do so—if it were not for the dance by which he externalizes the role. In embodying his self-criticism, I feel linked to his father. Like his father, I call him out for denying his role in indulging himself—then with his mother, now with his lovers.

We have fallen into this pattern before and I have interpreted it directly. He tends to be receptive to the notion that I can personify a self-critical voice that he learned from his father. He tends to assume, however, even after such interpretations, that the criticism is warranted. He protests his innocence as a defense against his conviction that he is an evil child. Instead of repeating the genetic interpretation, I offer a clarification. I explain that I am pointing out an *unconscious* pattern, not a conscious action plan. The clarification suggests an implicit compromise. I agree that he lacked awareness in the past. I implicitly forgive him for his unwitting actions and ask him to take responsibility in the present. He laughs a sheepish but, to my ears, genuine assent and re-iterates his progress.

A long pause follows. I linger silently over his comment that Skyler's ex has everything. He tends to be vague in his comments about other men. I imagine he uses vague language to defend himself against the painful articulation of what he feels he lacks. I wait for his next association. He seems to be waiting for me. I imagine that he would like me to ask about the comment—to challenge him to face and work through his envy.

I do ask. He tells me of a rival who is handsome, likable and on the cusp of a successful career in entertainment. He has Skyler in his power. She wants to fuck him—just to fuck him. He doesn't have to be nice, or to promise commitment. She just wants him.

He is insistent in his tone as if he feels the need to convince me. Perhaps he thinks I will refuse to recognize the inherent pleasure in being the object of a woman's lust. I explicitly recognize it *would* be validating. He elaborates. The male object of desire is a "fun attractive person"—a man Travis jealously disparages for "breaking the rules."

The fun, attractive man might represent the unseen character who stole his mother in childhood. He is, in this session and in general, portrayed as a performing artist or entertainer. I imagine Travis has retroactively filled in the outlines with his own ideal self-image. I want to open up this aspect of the imagery. I comment that it is usually an artist.

Travis articulates his image of the rival: a relaxed but playful bad-boy in hipper clothes. He sees himself, by contrast, as a polite dork, a jealous square. In his image, he is too afraid to play with fireworks. The other kids rush out to enjoy the display. The fireworks perhaps represent the phallic masculinity that he is too timid to let himself enjoy.

Second Session

Travis: I saw Jenna last night. She always has this blank expression. No matter what you do. You have no idea if she's having a good time, not having fun, indifferent, hating it, wanting to leave. You just don't know. There's no flirtation. We sat on opposite ends of the couch and got drunk. Then we went into my bedroom and had sex. I couldn't tell if she was enjoying it. At one point I stopped and was like, "Do you even like doing this?" "Yea," she said. Just, "Yea." There was just nothing getting me into it. I don't want to sleep with someone who feels nothing for me. After sex she just lay there without saying anything. I asked her again if she even liked doing it. She said, "We like to finish too you know." So that hurt. I just don't think she likes sleeping with me.

[Brief pause.]

Travis: Things have been really slow at work. I've been feeling bored. I keep thinking back to Lindsey. I keep wondering if she slept with Pete [his coworker]. My and Lindsey's friend Caleb is getting pretty huge [in the Indie music world]. I wonder how far the rumors have spread. I wonder if I really deserve them. I always feel like I don't belong. Why doesn't Jenna like having sex with me?

[Brief pause.]

Travis: I texted her to ask her directly. She said, "Yes. I already told you that." I don't buy it. I don't want her to think I'm pathetic. Here let me read it to you. [He takes out his phone]. I said, "I picture you rolling your eyes in boredom." She said, "I'm just trying to get choked and have my hair pulled to be honest." [He tosses the phone aside.] Great, one of those. Why does she need that? If sex is fulfilling some sort of psychological thing for her, I don't want to be a part of that. I'm not into rough sex. But a lot of guys are. But why should I care how masculine I am? Why do I need to play into some sort of stereotype? Why should I feel ashamed? I start to get really mad.

[He is visibly agitated. He takes a breath and lets his hands drop to the couch.]

Travis: I picture my sexually liberated friends. A lot of rock bands sing about that these days. I imagine my friends considering me a boring sex partner. I think being rough satisfies a weak part of the male psyche that needs to feel manly. It's the same part that makes guys spread their legs on the train. Why should I force that? I don't have that.

[Brief pause.]

Travis: But then maybe if she were more validating, I could get into that.

[Brief pause]

Travis: I try to console myself. I say to myself, "You put yourself in the role of an absolute loser, but she's not saying that." I try to let her confront me. I try to hear her confirmation. She is telling me that I read into it too much.

Greg: You fight yourself to feel that you could you have more worth—to her and to yourself.

Travis: I compare myself to other men. Even if it's not on the table, I'll find a way to do it.

[Brief pause]

Travis: But there's another thing about this too. I'm starting to be more honest—whether it's the right thing to say or not. Like saying, "I'm not really into that." I can't force myself to be something I'm not. But that's scary. I never know which feelings are correct. Maybe I'm not doing my job in bed. Or maybe I just don't like being rough. But I was that way with

Adrienne. It felt super-inspired. I don't know why. It's too big a topic to get into.

[Brief pause]

Travis: The thing is Jessica likes me. She tells me, and I don't fucking listen. Why don't I see the positive things she's giving me? Why do I need her to be more engaged?

Greg: The problem isn't that you need affirmation—that's just human. The problem is that you don't trust it when you get it. You don't trust it when Jenna says she likes you.

Travis: But if she likes me, then why is she so shy around me? She isn't like that around other guys.

Greg: That could mean many things. Maybe she likes you more. Maybe that's why she gets clammed up.

Travis: That is what happens! But why doesn't she treat me like other guys? You know she sleeps with some of them. Right away. Like, on the first date.

Greg: And you think it's because, on some visceral level, she's more attracted to them than she is to you.

Travis: That matters!

Greg: I don't disagree. You want her to choose you—at least in part—out of lust. But you feel inferior to those other guys. So you present yourself as the nice guy—the sensitive alternative. And guess what: You win. You get the girl. But you can't take any pleasure in it. You tell yourself she just defaulted to you out of safety or comfort. You can't shake the idea that she would prefer to be with some other guy. When she says she wants you to choke her—you, by the way, not someone else, not one of those other guys—you take it as a confirmation of your fear. As if it were impossible for you to be the gentle *and yet aggressive* guy who turns her on.

Travis: Yea.

[A few minutes of silence before session ends.]

Discussion

Travis spent the previous night with Jenna. He was disturbed by her blank facial expression. He could not tell if she was enjoying herself. He asks her explicitly, and she says, 'Yea.' He is put-off by her flat, one-word answer. After sex, he asks her again if she likes what they are doing. She replies in a patronizing way that women like to finish too. He ignores the explicit message that she would have liked *him* to bring her to an organism. (She is ostensibly frustrated that *he* did not let her finish.) Travis focuses instead on what he considers the subtext: that Jenna would rather be fucking someone else.

I wonder silently if her blank face evokes implicit memories of his mother's flat affect. He seems to fill the blank space in the woman's mind with the later developed image of a male rival. I do not have enough material for an interpretation and so keep listening.

He wonders aloud if Lindsey, an ex-girlfriend, slept with his current coworker Pete. When he was dating Lindsey, he in fact introduced her to Pete and a few other friends. Travis later accused her of being flirtatious with him. She said she was just being friendly. Travis often recalls the easy banter Lindsey and Pete shared. He convinces himself they met up later. He imagines them bad-mouthing him. From past sessions, I know he fears being portrayed as a jealous and possessive creep of mediocre talent. He imagines the rumors getting to the up-and-coming Caleb and spreading through the music scene. He acts as if it had already happened. He feels excluded from a world of peers who relate easily to each other. He implies it is unfair of them to ostracize him.

He now returns to his inadequacy in Jenna's eyes. He doubts her reassurance. He is certain she sees him as pathetic. He accuses her of being bored in their sex life. He shows me she wants him to be more dominant ("I'm just trying to get choked and have my hair pulled."). He then retreats in disgust. He complains she wants him to play into a stereotype. He implies he doesn't care how masculine he is. He suggests that behind her fantasy, there must be some perverse psychological need. He refuses to indulge her perversion. He thereby wins a cheap moral victory over the woman he feels inadequate for.

He expounds his ethical position. He tries to differentiate himself from what he portrays as a sex-obsessed music culture. To his sexually liberated friends, who are part of that world, he would, he imagines, come off as dull or boring in bed. But in rejecting their model, he rejects the male chauvinism he finds personified in men who spread their legs on the train. He asks me why he should force himself to be like them. It's a rhetorical question. He implies that he is better than them for rejecting their masculine display.

I imagine he is waiting for my applause. When I don't affirm him, he shifts in tone. If she were more validating, he could perhaps get into the role in her fantasy. He walks me through how he encourages himself. He tells himself that *he* is the one making himself out to be a loser. He challenges himself to hear her assertion that she sees him differently.

I affirm his self-confrontation. I elaborate that he is challenging himself to play with alternative possibilities in which he has more worth. It is implicit—but I have said before—that he finds safety in the loser role. It is riskier to let himself believe in his sex appeal.

He picks up on the defense interpretation and elaborates the danger. He admits he compares himself to other men. Up until recently, he pretended to be above such comparisons. The comparison implies competitive feelings, which, in turn, evoke anxiety. He retreats to his old position: that he cannot force himself to be something he's not. To force it is to lose a compensatory identity grounded in repudiating that kind of masculinity. It is, moreover, to admit his deficiency. But he seems to want to challenge himself. He remembers Adrienne inspired him to be more assertive in bed. Suddenly he stops. With each new assertion of masculine striving, he seems to encounter more intense anxiety.

He criticizes himself for rejecting her positive feedback. He then turns on his very need for affirmation ("Why do I need her to be more engaged?"). It the past, he has retreated from feelings of rejection into a defensive autonomous stance. I try to interrupt the defense. The problem, I say, is not that he needs affirmation, but that he does not trust it when he gets it. In doing so I signal that the work lies not in embracing a defensive autonomy, but in looking at how hard he finds it to trust a woman's interest in him.

He then asks what seems like a naïve question. "If she likes me, then why is she so shy around me?" She isn't shy around other guys, he points out. I feel the need to educate him. It is as if I must teach him the basics or else leave him guessing at a world he is hopelessly unable to read. (I present my feeling as countertransference data.) I suggest simply that a woman who likes him might find herself inhibited and thus seem shy.

He agrees with me, but then hints at a deeper interpretation. He tells me, with a certain wink and nod, that she sleeps with other guys right away . . . "Like, on the first date." I see the conclusion he wants me to draw: She is shy around him because she merely *likes* him. She wants to *fuck* them—she is so turned on she can hardly restrain herself. The problem, he shows me, is less his naiveté than his phallic narcissistic vulnerability.

I decide *not* to voice my full inference. In doing so, I mean to chase him out of his vague hints and insinuations, and challenge him to face his apparent fear in being more direct. To push him, I elaborate just a hint of what he has implied: that these other men are more sexually appealing than him. I leave it for him to articulate a more complete fantasy.

'That matters!' He says, as if in protest. He apparently believes I think it *shouldn't* matter. He implicitly sets me up as the moral representative of mutual love and devotion. It is as if I want him to transcend his base phallic impulses. I become the voice of the (in his mind) feminist morality he personified before. He struggles, via projection, to externalize and reject an ethic of loving monogamy that smothers his emergent phallic desire.

It might have been possible to reflect on the projection itself: "So you think I think it shouldn't matter." But with him such comments tended not to lead anywhere. He would typically restate his impression of my stance until I clarified my actual position. He needed access to my real thoughts and feelings to orient his own thoughts and feelings.

I choose, therefore, simply to brush off the projection and solidify a point just within his grasp. He wants to be the object of a woman's lust—like the aggressive men in his associations—but he feels inferior and so retreats into a feminized position: the sensitive guy.[3] He then turns around and uses his nice-guy credentials to get girls. He doesn't really give up the fight, therefore, but simply changes his strategy to emphasize his strength. He is successful in the sense that he does beat out other guys to win over his partner. Yet, when she asks him to be more dominant in bed, he can only hear her admitting that she would prefer someone else. What could have been an invitation to freer sex—and a sign he could take on a more dominant role—only reinforces his gender split. He cannot imagine being someone who is gentle in life *and yet* aggressive in the bedroom.

He agrees and lies in silence. He tends to do so when I have said a lot. He prefers to mull over his thoughts in private first. I want to hear his response, but the session is over.

Third Session

Travis: What if Lindsey is sleeping with my coworker? I asked a third coworker. He couldn't believe I was asking. He was like, "Are you serious right now? Man, that's some crazy shit." But I don't know. Is it?

[Brief pause.]

Travis: I've been feeling anxious about the new album. Maybe I'm working in the wrong paradigm. I feel depressed because I'm stuck at the café.

[Brief pause.]

Travis: I'm pissed because everything I was working on, like the studio work, has stopped. Normally I'll come in and say, "I shouldn't be doing music." Now the fact that I haven't been doing it is starting to speak to me. Like, "Should I be doing this?" I'm coming here to learn about myself and what I should be doing, and I feel no closer to it. Yesterday I drove myself nuts trying to fix one part of one song.

Greg: You know it's okay if you don't want to do music.

Travis: Wait, what? Where was that three years ago?

Greg: Three years ago, fear was blocking you. You weren't writing. You hadn't written anything in years. You had to overcome your fear to give it a fair chance. Now you are giving it a chance. You've written new songs, recorded them, learned how to mix them. Even though you say you aren't doing it . . . you are. So if in the end you don't enjoy it, then okay. At least you've learned that.

Travis: Well that sounds good. It makes it feel like a choice. There's something in my head that says, "Of course you're going to do it. What could be more fun?"

[Brief pause.]

Travis: The problem is . . . I've seen myself as having something great in me to get out. But maybe I need to change the game—to see it as a game where I still don't know what I want to do. Something I can enjoy and get better at. Then it won't be like the snake eating its tail. Because I got hung up on a particular version of success. Does that make sense?

Greg: Yea, you can redefine it in a more fluid, open-ended way . . . to break out of the confines of what you pictured as a young twenty-something.

Travis: Yea, Sayre is dating a comedian with this "you can't understand my genius" kind of thing going on. And I'm like, "Yea . . . Oh man . . . It's a painful place to be." Sayre works at a place that reviews records. There's this pile where they put the records people submit that are never going to get reviewed. She told me they put this guy's record in the pile. I guess her coworkers were teasing him. Like, "Hey, dude, so you made a comedy record! Awesome!" He's talking about moving to Europe where he thinks people will understand him.

[Brief pause.]

Travis: I used to want my record to be some great thing. It's a painful place to be. I can see all of the places where it falls short.

[Brief pause.]

Travis: But if I look at my music career more as a journey where the goal is to evolve—to break free of the mold I've made for myself—I might do better. I might enjoy it more.

[Brief pause.]

Travis: But I fall into a trap. Everything I'm doing is to serve this predefined image. Breaking up with Lindsey. Worrying what other people think of me. I'm afraid of them talking about me at a show.

Greg: You misrecognize your ambition as an unjustified arrogance. To yourself you become an arrogant nobody. Then you act out of your insecurity. You think that's all people see. And you're afraid they're right: that you're a joke. A self-deceived, mean-spirited putz. Like the way you see the comedian. That puts all the more pressure on you to succeed. You have to succeed to prove them and yourself wrong. But you get lost in the proof. You lose your pleasure in the work.

Travis: Yea. I need a step-by-step process. Otherwise I get lost in proving myself. And there's no fucking point.

Discussion

Travis returns to the question of whether Lindsey is sleeping with his coworker Pete. He asks a third coworker who calls him crazy. But Travis isn't convinced yet. He asks me if I think it's a crazy idea. He often polls me, among others, for feedback on his reality-testing. If enough of us agree he is being crazy, Travis tends to relent. To relent is not to abandon the 'crazy' belief. It is merely to suppress it in deference to the majority opinion.

I remain silent. In doing so, I imply that she might or might not be seeing Pete. I want to let Travis sort it out and, if he can tolerate it, to explore the insecurity behind the fantasy.

Travis turns to the album. Something about it feels off. He wonders if he is working in the 'wrong paradigm.' He slips from his self-doubt into feeling stuck at the café. The setback—whatever it is—seems to signify the futility of his creative endeavors.

I say nothing to reassure him. I want to avoid a split in which I comfort him, and he rejects me out of self-contempt. (I would then embody his need to be soothed and he his self-loathing.) I want to see if he will, instead, risk reassuring himself about the album. To fight his own self-rejecting attitude is, in essence, to face the vulnerability of hope.

He ups the ante in a moment of apparent self-reckoning. He suggests, in the spirit of facing a hard truth, that, if he can't make progress, perhaps it means he should quit music. Why chase a dream if he isn't cut out for it? I feel an unspoken invitation to confront him: "Is it true that you aren't making progress? Aren't you taking the setback too hard? Don't all artists face challenges? Isn't it more about perseverance than raw talent?" I check these thoughts. I am used to a certain bait-and-switch. He baits me into being an encouraging parent or mentor and then acts as if I am forcing him to keep striving. He thereby disavows his ambition and conveniently rejects it by rejecting my pressure.

I take a different and perhaps more honest tack. "You know it's okay if you don't want to do music." I convey (and mean it) that I will accept him whether or not he pursues music. I refuse to collude in his defensive maneuver to make me the success hungry parent. He must avow his own ambitions and pursue them (or not) on his own terms.[4]

He is startled. "Wait, what? Where was that three years ago?" For years I have indeed focused on his fear of pursuing artistic goals and his various means of defensive evasion. He has heard my effort at defense analysis as a tacit demand that he make good on his talent. I could not deny the grain of truth in his perception.[5] I *did* want him to overcome his fear sufficiently to give music a chance. He has, so many years later, used the analysis to work through much of his anxiety and so become more consistent in his creative work. If after giving it a fair chance, he no longer wants to be a musician, then he is free, as I tell him, to give it up. My wish was simply for him to try it and learn from experience.

The moment I relieve him of my pressure he rebounds. "Well that sounds good. It makes it feel like a choice. There's something in my head that says, 'Of course you're going to do it. What could be more fun?'" The sequence suggests that, when I refuse the role of task-master, he once again finds his own initiative. He can no longer isolate his ambition in me as a means of evading the danger implicit in letting himself want for more.

Travis elaborates on the danger. "The problem is . . . I've seen myself as having something great in me to get out." To invest in his great potential is, at this point, to suffer a loss. He has failed to realize "a version of success" forged in his teens and early twenties. He suggests reframing his project. "Maybe I need to change the game—to see it as a game where I still don't know what I want to do. Something I can enjoy and get better at." He challenges himself, in essence, to mourn his fantasy of early stardom and to adopt instead a process-goal—to enjoy the process of learning, cultivating and expressing himself.

He asks me if his reframe makes sense. He seems implicitly to ask if I accept his new goal. (Or if I see it—as he perhaps does in a more critical register—as a lame copout.) It makes sense, I affirm, to break the confines of what he pictured as a twenty-something.

He associates to an ex-girlfriend Sayre's new partner—a comedian with a "you can't understand my genius" attitude. Travis relates to the pain implicit in illusions of greatness. Sayre's coworkers mock this person, who believes (pathetically) that glory awaits him abroad. Travis links this man's comedy to his own album. "I used to want my record to be some great thing." To invest in it is to risk becoming a joke, like the comedian.

He then returns to his career reframe. He re-iterates that he might enjoy his musical pursuits more if he loosens prior images of success and focuses on the journey itself. He is prone, he repeats, to fall into a 'trap' in which he lives to serve a 'pre-defined image'—an image by which he has already failed. By repeating the session's interpretation, he seems to make it his own and to reinforce it against his implicit self-doubt.

I further articulate our co-constructed insight. I make explicit that he misrecognizes his ambition as unjustified arrogance. I do so to make space for healthy grandiose strivings. I suggest that he—like his father—misrecognizes such strivings as misguided arrogance. He then acts in a way, I say, that brings confirmation of his self-perception. He is then forced to prove his talent/worth. But in the process, he loses his enjoyment.

My aim is to clarify that he need not vilify his own ambition. I suspect that, if he can tolerate his ambition, instead of misrecognizing it as something to be hated, then he will find less need to act such a way as to make others dislike him and so externalize the feeling. He will fell less need to prove himself to them or to his imagined construction of them. He will then be freer to enjoy the artistic process (or to find that he does not enjoy it).

He again repeats the insight. "Yea. I need a step-by-step process. Otherwise I get lost in proving myself. And there's no fucking point." But he shies away from my later addition: the notion of healthy ambition. That particular idea is, I suspect, too fraught to consider.

Conceptualization

Defensive Regression

One might argue that Travis regressed defensively from phallic-phase castration anxiety to an anal organization (Cf. Freud, 1908, 1913a, 1917b, 1923, 1926; Jones, 1918; Abraham, 1923, 1924; Shengold, 1985; Chapter 9, pp. 178–183.) In the first session above, he arrives, after some digging, at his sense of inferiority vis-à-vis the 'kids' who play with 'fireworks'—perhaps a symbol of their orgasmic phallic potential. These kids/men—the lusty objects of female desire—have it all. He believes he will not have lived until he knows what it is like to be so hotly desired that women cannot suppress their appetite for him.

But to compete is to suffer inevitable humiliation—to become the pathetic comedian. He therefore regresses, the theory would suggest, to a more secure anal organization. In his imagery he becomes, in his imagery, a 'polite,' 'clean-cut' little boy. Such pleasure in obedience is thought to derive from toddler-age toilet training (Abraham, 1923). To be a good little boy is, moreover, by the logic of sphincter morality, to assert his superiority to the men who "spread their legs on the train" (Cf. Shengold, 1985). He thereby retreats into a compensatory moral victory over his phallic rivals.

To regress to anality is to revive the toddler's posited wish for passive anal stimulation (Freud, 1913a). The same wish later manifests, according to

Freud, in the homoerotic desire to be penetrated anally. In regressing, Travis might, then, revive his own wish to be penetrated by a phallic man. He perhaps projects his taboo craving onto women at large. In his mind, they wish to be penetrated just as he, in theory, wishes to be penetrated. The projection reinforces his belief that he cannot give them what he/they want.

Travis feels burdened, in the first two sessions, by thwarted fantasies of artistic success. In the third session, he attempts to re-focus his attention on the learning process itself. He seems to want me to validate this reframe. One might understand the reframe as a reinforcement of his anal defense. He retreats, in essence, from (phallic) creative production to (anal) mastery as an aim in itself. Such an interpretation assumes that the pleasure in mastery originates in anal sphincter control (Freud, 1905, p. 198). He pressures me, by this account, to affirm and so collude in his anal retreat from castration anxiety.

Restorative Regression

Beneath the anal presentation one might posit a primary longing to regress back into the pre-Oedipal mother (Cf. Ferenczi, 1938; Winnicott, 1965; Balint, 1968; Kohut, 1971). Such a longing might manifest in his hypersensitivity to lapses in his partner's attention. He begins, in typical fashion, by minimizing the degree of his dependency on women. ("I want a girlfriend, but nothing is working out, so I'm not thinking about it too much.") In the second session, he shows, however, how sensitive he is to his partner's affect. ("Jenna always has this blank expression. No matter what you do.") One is reminded of his early memories of boredom in his mother's presence. Perhaps he strives by phallic means to recreate an earlier—traumatically ruptured—sense of mother–infant union.

The patient in such a state often hears interpretations as 'something else' (Balint, 1968, p. 9). I interpret the defenses, for instance, by which Travis evades the anxiety in his creative work. I want to empower him to face the danger (regardless of the outcome). But he hears an implicit charge: to win my approval it is imperative that he succeed in his calling. A merger appears in which my desire absorbs his own and reproduces it as a demand.

He responds to clarifications by which I repair ruptures and restore his sense of control. I clarify, for instance, that it's okay if he gives up music. He is surprised. ("Wait, what? Where was that three years ago?"). I explain the purpose of defense analysis: not to make a demand, but to empower him to experiment and make his own decision. He feels a surge in initiative. ("Well that sounds good. It makes it feel like a choice. There's something in my head that says, 'Of course you're going to do it. What could be more fun?'") One might argue that, in repairing the rupture and following his initiative, I provide the mothering he seeks outside the room through constant sexual affairs.

He uses me, on this analysis, to provide the maternal care he needs, not for sexual gratification per se, but, much more fundamentally, to develop a sense of authentic selfhood, manifest, in this case, in the ability to say what he wants and make his own choices. The provision, which includes well-attuned interpretation, drives the therapeutic action.

Explanatory Gaps

The critique of regression *does not* require us to dismiss the plausibility of these early dynamics. It is quite possible that mother–infant ruptures *did* predispose him to seek maternal care through later sexual relationships. It is possible, moreover, that, sensing his inadequacy, he later retreated from male competition into a good-little-boy position. By this means, he avoided defeat and secured whatever female affection he could.

There are, however, several explanatory gaps in the above regression-based conceptualizations. We find, to begin, a lack of specificity. Travis pursues a specific female character (a muse) against a specific male rival (a more dominant male singer-songwriter). It would seem forced to derive their qualities solely from his mother and father. We shall require later development to understand the specific form taken by the conflict.

The above regression theories address early developmental anxieties. The first addresses castration anxiety; the second the fear of rupture in a transferential mother–infant bond. They do not recognize the *new* developmental anxieties of the young adult patient. We find his dread, for instance, at the possibility he is not the talent he thinks he is. He fears his entire identity might turn out to be a grandiose illusion. Such a danger presupposes the adolescent and young adult construction the artistic identity he fears losing.

The regression theories fail, lastly, to address the mourning process at play in the present developmental context. Travis has failed, by now, to realize an earlier dream of precocious success. To face the failure is to mourn the loss of a defining fantasy. Only by mourning the loss can he restore himself and dare to strive again toward a revised dream. It is not a return to anything, but a loss he faces only now upon entry into his thirties.

From the Logic of Regression to Progression

The two regression interpretations rely on separate, but potentially compatible, reconstructions of the patient's childhood. They posit a regression to that which has been reconstructed. The resulting formulation leaves open the three above gaps. The critique of regression does not discard the two reconstructions. It simply re-frames the regression as a progression. The patient *progresses* from childhood to here-and-now tasks and dangers.

The analysis of progression begins, like the regression analyses, in a reconstructed childhood. The transference and extra-transference data suggest (but cannot prove) that he did experience jarring moments of maternal misattunement. He is hyper-sensitive, for instance, to my slight misunderstandings. He is vulnerable, moreover, to his partner's blank affect. He feels pressure to become whatever I and/or she needs him to be to get recognition. He has no direct memories of his pre-Oedipal mother. We know only that she was so unstable, or appeared so unstable, that the father won full custody. Travis internalized her, in later memories, as alternately exciting (cotton-candy) and preoccupied (doing laundry in the other room). We can infer that, from a very young age, perhaps before his explicit memories, Travis sought to overcome her inconsistency and win her attention. He perhaps felt thwarted in a manner revived in his transference and dating life.

Travis presents only sparse material from the Oedipal years. He recalls pressure, from at least age five onwards, to side with his father against his mother. His father would, he recalls, rehearse the judge's custody ruling and do what he could to vilify his mother. According to his father, she did not really love her children. She put some third object—perhaps a man, perhaps drugs, perhaps her own lifestyle—above Travis and his sister.

We find here an early instance of deferred action. Travis, as mentioned, felt a mild boredom in his mother's presence. He drew on his father's portrait to flesh her out as an internal character. He felt bored *because* she neglected him *because* she didn't truly love him. From boredom he thus moves, via his father's story, to represent an internal mother with self-serving and supremely inconsiderate motives.

On weekend visitations, Travis nonetheless relished the one-on-one time with his mother. The cotton-candy story suggests a feeling of forbidden pleasure in their relationship. In the story, he must downplay a fun outing in order to placate his father's jealousy. Privately he wished he could go live with her. Perhaps he felt he had won the rivalry for his mother's affection. His father seemed to perceive and perhaps amplify the competition. He insisted Travis renounce his mother and accept him as the one true parent. Travis identified with his father. He later became the one to interrogate others, as his father had interrogated him, about their hidden infidelities and intention to abandon him.

In latency his father became—at least in Travis' recall—hyper-aggressive in his conduct. Travis was supposed to reject his mother and turn to receive his father's tough love. But as in the baseball story, he withdrew and refused to compete for paternal recognition. He was lonely and isolated—primed to look outside the home for alternative models.

He found alternatives in adolescence in a subgenre of melancholy Indie rock music. The men were slender, thoughtful and emotive. They represented a masculinity very different from his father's. In imitating them, Travis rejected his father and moved toward a new organizing fantasy. To establish himself among his idols was to defeat his father and, in fantasy, to win the universal love and adoration of which he had been deprived.

The adolescent fantasy of creative success reorganized the original Oedipal triangle. He transferred latent competitive feelings from his father to his creative peer rivals. The young muse, moreover, displaced his mother as the primary object of his desire. We learn about the original Oedipal conflict mostly by retroactive inference from the new organization.

We must understand his passive masculine presentation in the context of his identity formation. The anal regression theory would regard it as the symptom of a retreat from castration anxiety in the phallic phase to a passive, perhaps feminized, anal position. It is possible that he does indeed draw on past anal identifications. He does so not in a *regression*, however, but in a *progression* into an emergent gender identity. He rejects his male body (his muscles) and embraces a feminine identification (female song protagonists) not just to retreat from his father, but, more drastically, to leave his father's world and gain entry into a new realm in which he strives for separate success and recognition. It is a realm in which it is an achievement (not a failure) to be a feminine guy.

We find a second example of deferred action in his junior year. He briefly dates a girl who cheats on him. He suspects something and confronts her. At first she lies, but later admits it. He is enraged by her effort to gaslight him. In his anger he is reminded of a vague hint in his father's tone toward his mother. He 'realizes' that his father spoke out of a similar hurt place: His mother must have cheated. The deferred action fills out a blank space in his picture of his mother's life. In her preoccupation, she was thinking of another man. The new betrayal registers as a re-iteration of the 'original' maternal betrayal.

In his twenties Travis tried and, by his own lights, failed to realize his creative ambition. He was forced to mourn a teenage fantasy of precocious success. To mourn he must confront what he has internalized of his father's criticism: that he is a "whiny little brat" who just makes noise to get attention. He is inclined to interpret the immediate setback as a confirmation. The implication is suicidal: "I think I should just poison the brat."

The 'brat' character does not, however, reflect the direct reliving of a childhood configuration. It is, in essence, the name by which Travis personifies present grandiose strivings. The strivings—which originated in childhood—have entered into a fantasy of adult failure. Travis represents this fantasy in the third session in the figure of the comedian. The comedian is a self-deceived character who insists on his unrecognized greatness. Others mock him. Even his girlfriend finds him misguided. Meanwhile he plans his escape to a far-away place where he foolishly hopes the people will appreciate his talent. Travis fears that, unless he rejects his grandiose hopes, he will become this person.

The defensive regression and irreversible lifespan approaches view the comedian differently. The defensive regression analysis portrayed him as an infantile castration symbol. The irreversible lifespan analysis recognizes and incorporates the phallic valence in this image. Whatever might have been the little boy's castration fear, the danger has evolved, however, beyond its first iteration into a sophisticated fantasy with present psychosocial significance. The sophistication is manifest, in this instance, in the representation of a character who insists on his greatness against a creeping feeling of inadequacy and self-deception. Not until latency do children develop the implicit capacity to represent contradictory feeling states in the same character (Harter, 1986; Westen, 1989; Fischer & Ayoub, 1994). Later in adolescence the subject then brings such representational capacities, among other integrative functions, to bear on the task of imagining a social role and an implicit conception of identity failure (Erikson, 1950, 1968). The comedian is not, therefore, a direct representation of infantile castration anxiety. The image pulls any early castration anxiety forward into a progressively elaborated fantasy of what it would look like for a young man to fail in the world.

One problem of the regression analyses was their lack of specificity. A lifespan approach, by contrast, helps us see in greater detail how identity formation reconfigured his rivalries. Travis imagines himself in constant rivalry with more successful artists and performers. The rival artist characters reflect something of his earlier rivalry with his father. Like his father, they seem to have their heads on straight. They are less self-deceived. They are comfortable inhabiting a dominant masculinity Travis rejects but envies.

Not all of their significant qualities derive, however, from his father. In his imagination, they have tattoos, hip clothes and laid-back attitudes. They are so appealing, on a visceral level, that women cannot help but fall into bed with them. They go beyond his father in this sense to reflect an alternative male aesthetic that has captivated him since adolescence when he discovered in his magazines an alternative to his father's example. They represent his father only indirectly through the rock star Travis aspires to be.

We find a third instance of deferred action in Travis' infidelity. He had come to see himself as a loser incapable of sustaining a woman's interest. He expected women, like his internal mother, a product of deferred action, to abandon him for more exciting men. So, he began to cheat preemptively—normalizing the betrayal he anticipated. It so happened that many of his partners, whom he juggled simultaneously, believed in his fidelity. Their naïve belief in him only further reinforced that he would be a fool to trust them. He believed he had learned from his early mother not to trust in the affection of a woman. In truth he had re-interpreted her lapses in attention in light of later events, and now in light of his own psychology, to construct an internal mother who justified his actions. She—and women in general—were *like him* always on the prowl for something better.

We saw above how identity formation in adolescence reconfigured the rivalries in his psyche. So too did it shape his erotic desire. In what I shall call the 'muse'—an implicit character in the sessions—Travis brings the mother of deferred action into a feminine presence whom he needs to affirm his artistic strivings. We find different aspects of the muse in the various women who flit through his associations. Jenna, like his internal mother, finds him dull. She accepts his attention, out of apathy and boredom, while she waits for a real man. Sayre implicitly establishes herself, in her pity for her comedian boyfriend, as an arbiter of real talent. The women—as characters in his psyche—lust for real men who can inspire them to new heights. To command their attention is, in turn, to be confirmed in his worth. To serve as muse a woman must bring a certain aesthetic edge. (He rejects women who do not.) They bring the flightiness of his internal mother into a new character who mirrors his search for an identity in artistic production.[6]

To come full circle, we might reframe the posited regression as a shift from rivalry to merger. The rivals were not direct representations of his childhood father, but brought certain of his qualities, for example, his masculinity, his reality-testing, forwards into a new character—the peer artist who personified Travis search for an identity beyond the family. He retreated from rivalry with them, and perhaps unconsciously with the analyst, into a merger in which he drew on my affirmation and belief in his worth to sustain his confidence. It was a 'merger' in the sense that my belief in him became his belief in himself. (By the term I do not imply a literal perceptual blurring of the skin-to-skin boundary.) But with whom was he merged? I seemed an amalgamation of past and present influences. I perhaps represented the maternal nurturance and consistency he longed for in childhood. At the same time, I might have represented something of his early father. Like his father, I became, for instance, the arbiter of reality/distortion. He left it up to me whether or not he should give up music, whether or not he should trust a given girlfriend etc. I brought these qualities forwards into a voice that personified his search for identity. I demanded—at least in his mind—that he become a musician. I refused to let him give up on his dream. In this regard I became—like the peer rivals and female muses—a *contemporary* object who brought past influences forwards into a new character.

When I met Travis, he was almost thirty and not yet famous. He faced a new—and devastating—task: to find worth and accept love even though he had not achieved his dream. Together we analyzed his retreat from creative ambition. Implicitly I showed my belief in his potential—a belief he could draw upon to bolster his nascent belief in himself. He became more consistent in his artistic output. To the extent that his process-oriented reframe was an anal defense (see Session 3), it was also a forward-striving adaptation. It enabled him to engage in work without clinging to past images of fame and glory. He began to trust, though tentatively, in his future appeal for a reliable and inspired woman. Implicitly, he was tasked to mourn a fantasy of redemption through early success. Very slowly, he grew to imagine himself as a viable person with something to offer.

Notes

1 A shorter version of this case has been accepted for publication in *The Psychoanalytic Study of the Child* (Rizzolo, in press at time of writing). Reprinted by permission of the journal and Yale University Press.

2 Blos (1967) argued, as previously mentioned, that the adolescent regresses "in self-contrived confrontations with miniature editions or proxy representations of the original [childhood] trauma" in order to master "prototypical danger situations" (p. 172). Travis, though in his thirties, provides a good example. He deliberately sought a love triangle, reminiscent of his early family situation, in which he would feel betrayed by a woman. He did so in order to master his jealousy. But, as argued above, and as is implicit in Blos' language, the new "proxy" is not a direct reliving—not a literal return to an earlier psychological state. He enters the new triangle, aware of how much his jealousy has ruined for him, with a recognition and a purposefulness he did not have in childhood.

3 I do not mean that to be "nice" or "sensitive" is to be feminine in any gender-essentialist sense. A man can, of course, embody such qualities without turning into a woman. I use these categories as they operate in his usage.

4 In the past, I tried to play the role, or contain the projection, in the spirit of reflection. "You feel I want you to pursue music." At other times, I would observe the bait-and-switch. "You seem to want my encouragement, but you are quick to feel that I'm pushing too hard, like I want it more than you do, like I won't accept you if you give up." He lacked a certain as-if capacity to play with the role he put me in. The above comments tended to reinforce his criticism. In the end he wanted to know—in a literal sense—why I was apparently so hell-bent on his musical success.

5 I had previously tried, as elaborated in endnote 3, to explore the role he assigned me. He tended, as mentioned, to hear my invitation to explore as a round-about confession that I had, in fact, put unreasonable demands on him. He was acutely sensitive, moreover, to being invalidated in his sense of reality. Behind his sensitivity, he tended actively to discredit himself—an aftereffect of his father's interrogations. I tried, as a matter of principle, to avow, or at least consider, the potential truth in his perception as prerequisite for any subsequent exploration. I wanted to establish, against his tendency to discredit himself, that he had the capacity to form a valid opinion.

6 Before he can handle mutual intimacy—the capacity for mutual surrender, devotion and generosity—the person loves out of a "self-seeking," "identity-hungry" impulse (Erikson, 1968, p. 137). Through the other, he hopes to find himself. Travis exemplified such self-seeking love. The ideal woman was, by and large, an extension of his pursuit.

Chapter 11

Conclusion

I have argued against traditional regression theories that the person—the irreducible subject of psychoanalytic inquiry—is inextricably embedded in the developmental present. We can reframe so-called regressions as shifts between motives, defenses and emotional states, each of which emerges out of a lifespan of growth. The adult analysand shifts between positions, sometimes to evade, sometimes to confront the tasks and anxieties at play in the here-and-now. He does not return, because no one can return, to the psychological condition of childhood in which his problems originated. The work of development is, in this regard, the work of mourning what is lost forever.

The argument began in the defensive and restorative traditions of regression. The first tradition frames regression as a retreat from new developmental anxiety to an earlier position of security. Behind any such regression, the second tradition posits a primary (non-defensive) pull to relax back into the nourishing environment of the infant–parent dyad. Both traditions yield intricate and nuanced approaches to the dynamics of human suffering. The task, for any critique of regression, is to preserve their insight in a revised model by which we can gain a more complete, and less infantilizing, picture of the adult patient.

I considered two traditions of critique: the conservative and radical critiques of regression. The conservative critique aims to clarify the term and to ensure its proper application. One key strategy is to portray the person as a machine with mature and regressed parts. The radical critique suggests, by contrast, that the term is irredeemably flawed. It inevitably perpetuates a genetic fallacy and, behind it, a defensive morality of maturity.

We should, by implication, discard the concept for a more nuanced lifespan approach.

This project aims, in short, to flesh out a model in which we can discard the regression concept. The first step, I have argued, is to set up the person as the irreducible subject of psychoanalytic inquiry. The irreducibility of the person rules out the above machine strategy. The person—who always acts out of the totality of the lifespan—is the one who operates the figurative gears. He operates even the most childish ones. To understand his actions—even the most childlike actions—we must understand his life history.

The person acts and makes sense of his action in the here-and-now relational field. He cannot regress *because* the immediate field infuses and reconfigures his internal world. The most rudimentary mechanism of growth here is deferred action. Through deferred action, he transcribes, and re-transcribes, the internalizations of earlier development. He thereby revises and updates his internal world in light of his immediate context.

I attempt to situate the field in a lifespan model of development. The person evolves—even in the deepest layers of unconscious—through each successive phase of life. To make this case, we must reject Freud's (1915) second sense of timelessness. The unconscious does, contrary to the second sense, develop through a lifelong history of influences. The mechanism of growth, once again, is deferred action. The person re-constellates his internal world amidst the tasks and anxieties of each new phase. We find psychopathology not in regression but in the rigidity by which he perpetuates historical problems.

By regression some analysts mean not a literal return to an earlier developmental phase, but, remaining within the present life phase, a retreat to primitive phantasies and defenses. The term *primitive* originated in the Freudian/Kleinian equation: regressed analysand = normative child = third-world subject = primitive subject. But the so-called primitive processes—namely, hallucinatory gratification, condensation, splitting and projective identification—are not intrinsically primary in human evolution or development. They develop, as I have shown, from rudimentary infantile to sophisticated adult forms. To enlist them is not to regress, but to rely on increasingly complex mental operations. The critique of regression applies equally, then, to this particular use of the term.

There has been a growing emphasis, across schools, on the analysis of the here-and-now (e.g., Joseph, 1978, 1989, 2013; Gill, 1979, 1984b;

Sandler & Sandler, 1984, 1987, 1994a). Despite their differences the proponents believe that genetic interpretation stems from, and is only useful in so far as it illuminates, the more immediate analysis of present dynamics. The critique of regression reinforces that the analysis of the present is depth work. Only in the here-and-now field does the person bring his deep motives to bear on his life. Genetic interpretation does not lead deeper into the unconscious. It is a here-and-now narrative activity. As such it reflects and extends the analysis of present tensions.

To illustrate the critique of regression in practice I have presented three analytic cases. In the first case we find a man who grew to identify with his father's violent impulsivity. He developed crippling obsessional defenses from adolescence onwards to defend against what he unconsciously recognized, I argue, as his emergent potential to cause real harm. The second case presents a man who similarly identified with a domineering mother and abusive father to become a sexual sadist who delighted in humiliating his objects. The third case describes a man who progressed from a rivalry with his father for a preoccupied mother to a search for identity that reproduced both parents in his own image. In each case the central dynamics originated in childhood. We require a lifespan analysis, however, to explain the progression from childhood to their respective adult presentations.

In presenting the cases, I propose a methodology that can be extended into future research. The method addresses the psychoanalytic problem of the non-risky depth hypothesis. Regression theorists tend, as I have argued, to offer non-risky hypotheses. They are non-risky because they pertain to unobservable unconscious processes. The regression proponent can always argue that, beneath the empirical analytic process, there is an unconscious infantile impulse, one too deep to be seen, that generates the empirical data. What data could ever invalidate the possibility of such an impulse beneath the data itself?

The best way to critique a regression hypothesis is not to challenge its reconstruction of the patient's childhood, but to show that, no matter how plausible its reconstruction, it leads to an *incomplete* understanding unless one proceeds to account for later development. To show its incompleteness one must first articulate what one would expect to observe if the patient had, in fact, regressed the childhood phase or stage in question. One must then show that the analytic process *disconfirms* the regression-specific expectations. Perhaps the process disconfirms them because the reconstruction is flawed. It is often possible, to show, however, that it disconfirms them, not necessarily because the reconstruction is flawed, but because the process reflects the internalizations of later development. The most complete conceptualization—the one that best accounts for the observable analytic process—will always be, if the present critique stands, a lifespan interpretation.

References

Abraham, K. (1923). Contributions to the theory of the anal character. *International Journal of Psychoanalysis*. 4:400–418.

Abraham, K. (1924). A short study of the development of the libido, viewed in light of mental disorders. In *Selected Papers on Psychoanalysis*. London: The Hogarth Press, 1949, pp. 418–501.

Altman, N. (1993). Psychoanalysis and the urban poor. *Psychoanalytic Dialogues*. 3:29–49.

Altman, N. (2000). Black and white thinking: A psychoanalyst reconsiders race. *Psychoanalytic Dialogues*. 10:589–605.

Arlow, J., & Brenner, C. (1964). *Psychoanalytic Concepts and the Structural Theory*. New York: International Universities Press.

Aron, L. (1991). The patient's experience of the analyst's subjectivity. *Psychoanalytic Dialogues*. 1:29–51.

Aron, L. (1996). *A Meeting of Minds: Mutuality in Psychoanalysis*. Hillsdale, NJ: Analytic Press.

Balint, M. (1959). *Thrills and Regressions*. London: Karnac.

Balint, M. (1965). *Primary Love and Psychoanalytic Technique*. London: Tavistock Publications.

Balint, M. (1968). *The Basic Fault: Therapeutic Aspects of Regression*. Evantson: Northwestern University Press.

Baranger, M., & Baranger, W. (1964). "Insight" in the analytic situation. In: L.G. Fiorini (Ed.), *The Work of Confluence: Listening and Interpreting in the Psychoanalytic Field*. London: Karnac, 2009, pp. 1–15.

BCPSG. (2007). The foundational level of psychodynamic meaning: Implicit process in relation to conflict, defense and the dynamic unconscious. *International Journal of Psychoanalysis*. 88:843–860.

Beebe, B. (1986), Mother-infant mutual influence and the precursors of self and object representations. In J. Masling (Ed.), *Empirical Studies of Psychoanalytic Theories, vol. 2*. Hillsdale, NJ: The Analytic Press, pp. 27–48.

Benedek, T. (1959). Parenthood as a developmental phase—A contribution to the libido theory. *Journal of the American Psychoanalytic Association*. 7:389–417.

Bion, W. (1961). *Experiences in Groups and Other Papers*. New York: Routledge.

Bion, W. (1962). *Learning from Experience*. New York: Routledge.

Blass, R.B. (2011). On the immediacy of unconscious truth: Understanding Betty Joseph's 'here and now' through comparison with alternative views of it outside of and within Kleinian Thinking. *The International Journal of Psychoanalysis.* 92:1137–1157.
Blass, R.B. (2015). Conceptualizing splitting: On the different meanings of splitting and their implications for the understanding of the person and the analytic process. *International Journal of Psychoanalysis.* 96:123–139.
Blos, P. (1967). The second individuation process of adolescence. *Psychoanalytic Study of the Child.* 22:162–186.
Blum, H.P. (1983). The position and value of extratransference interpretation. *Journal of the American Psychoanalytic Association.* 31:587–617.
Boas, F. (1928). *Anthropology and Modern Life.* New York: Dover Publications.
Bollas, C. (1979). The transformational object. *International Journal of Psychoanalysis,* 60:97–107.
Bornstein, B. (1951). On latency. *Psychoanalytic Study of the Child.* 6:279–285.
Brickman, C. (2003). *Aboriginal Populations in the Mind.* New York: Columbia University Press.
Britton, R. (1992). The Oedipus situation and the depressive position. *New Library of Psychoanalysis.* 14:34–45.
Bromberg, P.M. (1996). Standing in the spaces: The multiplicity of self and the psychoanalytic relationship. *Contemporary Psychoanalysis.* 32:509–535.
Broughton, J. (1980). The divided self in adolescence. *Human Development.* 24:13–32.
Carey, S. (1985). *Conceptual Change in Childhood.* Cambridge, MA: MIT Press.
Coen, S.J. (2000). The wish to regress in patient and analyst. *Journal of the American Psychoanalytic Association.* 48:785–810.
Cole, M., & Scribner, S. (1974). *Culture and Thought: A Psychological Introduction.* New York: John Wiley & Sons.
Comte, A. (1830). *Introduction to Positive Philosophy.* Indianapolis: Hackett, 1988.
Davies, J.M. (1996). Linking the "pre-analytic" with the postclassical: Integration, dissociation, and the multiplicity of unconscious process. *Contemporary Psychoanalysis.* 32:553–576.
Davies, J.M., & Frawley, M.G. (1991). Dissociative processes and transference-countertransference paradigms in the psychoanalytically oriented treatment of adult survivors of childhood sexual abuse. In: S.A. Mitchell & L. Aron (Eds.), *Relational Psychoanalysis: The Emergence of a Tradition, Volume 14,* 1999. New York: Routledge, pp. 269–304.
Donee, L.H. (1973, March). *Infants' development scanning patterns of face and non-face stimuli under various auditory conditions.* Paper presented at the Meeting of the Society for Research in Child Development, Philadelphia, PA.
Edelman, J. (1987). *Neural Darwinism.* New York: Basic Books.
Erikson, E. (1950). *Childhood and Society.* New York: W. W. Norton & Company.
Erikson, E. (1958). *Young Man Luther.* New York: W. W. Norton & Company.
Erikson, E. (1968). *Identity: Youth and Crisis.* New York: W. W. Norton & Company.
Erreich, A. (2003). A modest proposal: (Re)defining unconscious fantasy. *Psychoanalytic Quarterly.* 72:541–574.
Faimberg, H. (2007). A plea for a broader concept of *Nachtraglichkeit. Psychoanalytic Quarterly.* 76:1221–1240.
Fairbairn, W.D. (1940). Schizoid factors in the personality. In: *Psychoanalytic Studies of the Personality,* 1952. London: Tavistock Publications, pp. 3–27.

Fairbairn, W.D. (1941). A revised psychopathology of the psychoses and psychoneuroses. In: David E. Scharff, MD & Ellinor Fairbairn Birtles (Eds.), *Psychoanalytic Studies of the Personality*, 1952. London: Tavistock Publications, pp. 28–58.

Fairbairn, W.D. (1952). In: David E. Scharff, MD & Ellinor Fairbairn Birtles (Eds.), *Psychoanalytic Studies of the Personality*. London: Tavistock Publications.

Feldman, M. (2009). Splitting and projective identification. In: B. Joseph (Ed.), *Doubt, Conviction and the Analytic Process*. New York: Routledge, 21–23.

Ferenczi, S. (1938/1989). *Thalassa: A Theory of Genitality*. London: Karnac.

Ferenczi, S., & Rank, O. (1925/2012). *The Development of Psychoanalysis*. Eastford, CT: Martino Fine Books.

Ferro, A. (1999a). *The Bi-Personal Field*. New York: Routledge.

Ferro, A. (1999b). *Psychoanalysis as Therapy and Storytelling*. New York: Routledge.

Ferro, A. (2002). *In the Analyst's Consulting Room*. New York: Routledge.

Fischer, K. (1980). A theory of cognitive development: The control and construction of hierarchies of skills. *Psychological Review*. 87(6):477–531.

Fischer, K., & Ayoub, C. (1994). Affective splitting and dissociation in normal and maltreated children: Developmental pathways for self in relationships. In: D. Cicchetti & S. Toth (Eds.), *Rochester Symposium on Developmental Psychopathology, Vol. 5: Disorders and Dysfunctions of the Self*. Rochester: University of Rochester Press, pp. 149–221.

Frazer, J.G. (1910). *Totemism and Exogamy: A Treatise on Certain Early Forms of Superstition and Society*. London: Macmillan.

Frazer, J.G. (1911–1915). *The Golden Bough: A Study in Magic and Religion*. 12 Volumes. London: Macmillan.

Freud, A. (1936/1966). *The Ego and the Mechanisms of Defense*. Madison, CT: International Universities Press.

Freud, A. (1965). *Normality and Pathology in Childhood: Assessments of Development*. New York: International Universities Press.

Freud, S. (1874). Letter from Sigmund Freud to Eduard Silberstein, December 20, 1874. The Letters of Sigmund Freud to Eduard Silberstein 1871–1881, 79–80.

Freud, S. (1875). Letter from Sigmund Freud to Eduard Silberstein, March 7, 1875. The Letters of Sigmund Freud to Eduard Silberstein 1871–1881, 94–99.

Freud, S. (1884). Uber coca. *Centrallblatt fur die ges Therapie*. 2:289–314. [Trans.: (abbreviated) Coca, *Saint Louis Medical Surgery Journal*, 47:502.]

Freud, S. (1900). *The Interpretation of Dreams*. The Standard Edition of the Complete Psychological Works of Sigmund Freud, Volume IV (1900): The Interpretation of Dreams (First Part), ix–627.

Freud, S. (1905). *Three Essays on the Theory of Sexuality* (1905). The Standard Edition of the Complete Psychological Works of Sigmund Freud, Volume VII (1901–1905): A Case of Hysteria, Three Essays on Sexuality and Other Works, 123–246.

Freud, S. (1908). *Character and Anal Erotism*. The Standard Edition of the Complete Psychological Works of Sigmund Freud, Volume IX (1906–1908): Jensen's 'Gradiva' and Other Works, 167–176.

Freud, S. (1909). *Notes Upon a Case of Obsessional Neurosis*. The Standard Edition of the Complete Psychological Works of Sigmund Freud, Volume X (1909): Two Case Histories ('Little Hans' and the 'Rat Man'), 151–318.

Freud, S. (1911). *Formulations on the Two Principles of Mental Functioning*. The Standard Edition of the Complete Psychological Works of Sigmund Freud, Volume XII (1911–1913): The Case of Schreber, Papers on Technique and Other Works, 213–226.

Freud, S. (1912). *The Dynamics of Transference*. The Standard Edition of the Complete Psychological Works of Sigmund Freud, Volume XII (1911–1913): The Case of Schreber, Papers on Technique and Other Works, 97–108.

Freud, S. (1913a). *The Disposition to Obsessional Neurosis, a Contribution to the Problem of the Choice of Neurosis*. The Standard Edition of the Complete Psychological Works of Sigmund Freud, Volume XII (1911–1913): The Case of Schreber, Papers on Technique and Other Works, 311–326.

Freud, S. (1913b). *Totem and Taboo: Some Points of Agreement between the Mental Lives of Savages and Neurotics* (1912–1913). The Standard Edition of the Complete Psychological Works of Sigmund Freud, Volume XIII (1913–1914): Totem and Taboo and Other Works, vii–162.

Freud, S. (1914). *On Narcissism: An Introduction*. The Standard Edition of the Complete Psychological Works of Sigmund Freud, Volume XIV (1914–1916): On the History of the Psycho-Analytic Movement, Papers on Metapsychology and Other Works, 67–102.

Freud, S. (1915a). *The Unconscious*. The Standard Edition of the Complete Psychological Works of Sigmund Freud, Volume XIV (1914–1916): On the History of the Psycho-Analytic Movement, Papers on Metapsychology and Other Works, 159–215.

Freud, S. (1915b). Overview of the transference neuroses. In: I. Grubrich-Simitis (Ed.), Hoffer & P. Hoffer (Trans.), *A Phylogenetic Fantasy: Overview of the Transference Neuroses*, Cambridge, MA: Harvard University Press, 1987.

Freud, S. (1917a). *Introductory Lectures on Psycho-Analysis*. The Standard Edition of the Complete Psychological Works of Sigmund Freud, Volume XVI (1916–1917): Introductory Lectures on Psycho-Analysis (Part III), 241–463.

Freud, S. (1917b). *On Transformations of Instinct as Exemplified in Anal Erotism*. The Standard Edition of the Complete Psychological Works of Sigmund Freud, Volume XVII (1917–1919): An Infantile Neurosis and Other Works, 125–134.

Freud, S. (1917c). *Mourning and Melancholia*. The Standard Edition of the Complete Psychological Works of Sigmund Freud, Volume VIV (1914–1916): On the History of the Psycho-Analytic Movement, Papers on Metapsychology and Other Works, 237–258.

Freud, S. (1918). *From the History of an Infantile Neurosis*. The Standard Edition of the Complete Psychological Works of Sigmund Freud, Volume XVII (1917–1919): An Infantile Neurosis and Other Works, 1–124.

Freud, S. (1920). *Beyond the Pleasure Principle*. The Standard Edition of the Complete Psychological Works of Sigmund Freud, Volume XVIII (1920–1922): Beyond the Pleasure Principle, Group Psychology and Other Works, 1–64.

Freud, S. (1921). *Group Psychology and the Analysis of the Ego*. The Standard Edition of the Complete Psychological Works of Sigmund Freud, Volume XVIII (1920–1922): Beyond the Pleasure Principle, Group Psychology and Other Works, 65–144.

Freud, S. (1923). *The Ego and the Id*. The Standard Edition of the Complete Psychological Works of Sigmund Freud, Volume XIX (1923–1925): The Ego and the Id and Other Works, 1–66.

Freud, S. (1924). *The Dissolution of the Oedipus Complex*. The Standard Edition of the Complete Psychological Works of Sigmund Freud, Volume XIX (1923–1925): The Ego and the Id and Other Works, 171–180.

Freud, S. (1926). *Inhibitions, Symptoms and Anxiety*. The Standard Edition of the Complete Psychological Works of Sigmund Freud, Volume XX (1925–1926): An Autobiographical

Study, Inhibitions, Symptoms and Anxiety, the Question of Lay Analysis and Other Works, 75–176.

Freud, S. (1930). *Civilization and its Discontents.* The Standard Edition of the Complete Psychological Works of Sigmund Freud, Volume XXI (1927–1931): The Future of an Illusion, Civilization and its Discontents, and Other Works, 57–146.

Freud, S. (1937a). *Analysis Terminable and Interminable.* The Standard Edition of the Complete Psychological Works of Sigmund Freud, Volume XXIII (1937–1939): Moses and Monotheism, An Outline of Psycho-Analysis and Other Works, 209–254.

Freud, S. (1937b). *Constructions in Analysis.* The Standard Edition of the Complete Psychological Works of Sigmund Freud, Volume XXIII (1937–1939): Moses and Monotheism, An Outline of Psycho-Analysis and Other Works, 255–270.

Freud, S., & Breuer, J. (1893–95). *Studies on Hysteria.* The Standard Edition of the Complete Psychological Works of Sigmund Freud, Volume II (1893–1895): Studies on Hysteria, v–323.

Fromm, E. (1991). Causes for the patient's change in analytic treatment. *Contemporary Psychoanalysis.* 27:581–601.

Gadamer, H.G. (1960). *Truth and Method,* trans. J. Weinsheimer & D.G. Marshall. New York: Continuum, 2003.

Galatzer-Levy, R.M. (1995). Psychoanalysis and dynamical systems theory: Prediction and self similarity. *Journal of the American Psychoanalytic Association.* 43:1085–1113.

Galatzer-Levy, R.M. (2002). Emergence. *Psychoanalytic Inquiry.* 22:708–727.

Galatzer-Levy, R.M. (2004). Chaotic possibilities: Toward a new model of development. *International Journal of Psychoanalysis,* 85:419–441.

Galatzer-Levy, R.M. (2009). Good vibrations: Analytic process as coupled oscillations. *International Journal of Psychoanalysis,* 90:983–1007.

Galatzer-Levy, R.M., & Cohler, B. (1993). *The Essential Other: A Developmental Psychology of the Self.* New York: Basic Books.

Gedo, J. (1979). Beyond Interpretation: Toward a Revised Theory for Psychoanalysis. New York: International Universities Press.

Gergely, G., & Watson, J.S. (1996). The social biofeedback theory of parental affect-mirroring. *International Journal of Psychoanalysis.* 77:181–1212.

Gerson, S. (2004). The relational unconscious: A core element of intersubjectivity, thirdness, and clinical process. *Psychoanalytic Quarterly.* 73:63–98.

Gertz, C. (1973). *The Interpretation of Cultures.* New York: Basic Books.

Ghent, E. (1990). Masochism, submission, surrender: Masochism as a perversion of surrender. *Contemporary Psychoanalysis,* 11:161–179.

Gill, M.M. (1954). Psychoanalysis and exploratory psychotherapy. *Journal of the American Psychoanalytic Association.* 2:771–797.

Gill, M.M. (1979). The analysis of transference. *Journal of the American Psychoanalytic Association.* 27S:263–288.

Gill, M.M. (1983). The point of view of psychoanalysis: Energy discharge or person? *Psychoanalysis and Contemporary Thought.* 6:523–551.

Gill, M.M. (1984a). Psychoanalysis and psychotherapy: A revision. *International Review of Psychoanalysis.* 11:161–179.

Gill, M.M. (1984b). Transference: A change in conception or only in emphasis? *Psychoanalytic Inquiry.* 4:489–523.

Gould, S.J. (1977). *Ontogeny and Phylogeny.* Cambridge, MA: Harvard University Press.

Greatrex, T.S. (2002). Projective identification: How does it work? *Neuropsychoanalysis*. 4:187–197.

Greenberg, J. & Mitchell, S.A. (1983) *Object Relations in Psychoanalytic Theory*. Cambridge, MA: Harvard University Press.

Greenson, R.R. (1965). The working alliance and the transference neurosis. *The Psychoanalytic Quarterly*. 34:155–181.

Grossmark, R. (2012). The unobtrusive relational analyst. *Psychoanalytic Dialogues*. 22:629–646.

Grunbaum, A. (1984). *The Foundations of Psychoanalysis: A Philosophical Critique*. Berkeley: University of California Press.

Habermas, J. (1968) *Knowledge and Human Interests*, trans. J.J. Shapiro, Boston: Beacon Press, 1972.

Haft, J. (2005). "On my way here I passed a man with a scab": Understanding a case of severe obsessive-compulsive disorder. *The Psychoanalytic Quarterly*. 74:1101–1126.

Harter, S. (1986). Cognitive-developmental processes in the integration of concepts about emotions and the self. *Social Cognition*. 4:119–151.

Harter, S., & Monsour, A. (1992). Developmental analysis of conflict caused by opposing attributes in the adolescent self-portrait. *Developmental Psychology*. 28:251–260.

Hartmann, H. (1939). *Ego Psychology and the Problems of Adaptation*. New York: International Universities Press.

Hartmann, H. (1955). Notes on the theory of sublimation. In: *Essays on Ego Psychology: Selected Problems in Psychoanalytic Theory*. New York: International Universities Press, 1964, pp. 215–240.

Hartmann, H., Kris, E., & Loewenstein, R.M. (1946). Comments on the formation of psychic structure. *Psychoanalytic Study of the Child*. 2:11–38.

Heidegger, M. (1927). *Being and Time*, trans. J. Macquarrie & E. Robinson. New York: Harper & Row, 1962.

Hinshelwood, R.D. (1991). *A Dictionary of Kleinian Thought*. Northvale, NJ: Jason Aronson.

Hinshelwood, R.D. (2008). Repression and splitting: Towards a method of conceptual comparison. *International Journal of Psychoanalysis*. 89:503–521.

Hinshelwood, R.D. (2013). *Research on the Couch: Single-Case Studies, Subjectivity and Psychoanalytic Knowledge*. New York: Routledge.

Hoffman, I.Z. (1983). The patient as interpreter of the analyst's experience. *Contemporary Psychoanalysis*. 19:389–422.

Hoffman, I.Z. (1991). Discussion: Toward a social-constructivist view of the psychoanalytic situation. *Psychoanalytic Dialogues*. 1:74–105.

Hoffman, I.Z. (1992). Some practical implications of a social-constructivist view of the psychoanalytic situation. *Psychoanalytic Dialogues*. 2:287–304.

Hoffman, I.Z. (1994). Dialectical thinking and therapeutic action in the psychoanalytic process. *Psychoanalytic Quarterly*. 63:187–218.

Inderbitzin, L.B., Levy, S.T. (2000). Regression and psychoanalytic technique: The concretization of a concept. *Psychoanalytic Quarterly*. 69:195–223.

Jacobson, E. (1964). *The Self and the Object World*. New York: International Universities Press.

Jones, E. (1918). Anal-erotic character traits. In: *Papers on Psychoanalysis*, Fifth Edition, 1949. Baltimore: The Williams and Wilkins Company.

Joseph, B. (1978). Different types of anxiety and their handling in the analytic situation. *International Journal of Psychoanalysis*. 59:223–228.

Joseph, B. (1985). Transference: the total situation. In: M. Feldman & E.B. Spillius (Eds.), *Psychic Equilibrium and Psychic Change: Selected Papers of Betty Joseph*. New York: Routledge, 1989, pp. 156–167.

Joseph, B. (1989). Psychic change and the psychoanalytic process. In: M. Feldman & E.B. Spillius (Eds.), *Psychic Equilibrium and Psychic Change: Selected Papers of Betty Joseph*. New York: Routledge, pp. 192–202.

Joseph, B. (2013). Here and now: My perspective. *International Journal of Psychoanalysis*. 94:1–5.

Katz, M.S. (2017). *Contemporary Psychoanalytic Field Theory: Stories, Dreams, and Metaphor*. New York: Routledge.

Kernberg, O. (1976). *Borderline Conditions and Pathological Narcissism*. New York: Jason Aronson.

Khun, T. (1962). *The Structure of Scientific Revolutions*. Chicago: University of Chicago Press.

Klein, M. (1927). Criminal tendencies in normal children. In: R. Money-Kyrle (Ed.), *Love, Guilt and Reparation and Other Works, 1921–1945*. New York: The Free Press, 1975, pp. 170–185.

Klein, M. (1928). Early stages of the Oedipus conflict. In: R. Money-Kyrle (Ed.), *Love, Guilt and Reparation and Other Works, 1921–1945*. New York: The Free Press, 1975, pp. 186–198.

Klein, M. (1930). The importance of symbol-formation in the development of the ego. In: R. Money-Kyrle (Ed.), *Love, Guilt and Reparation and Other Works, 1921–1945*. New York: The Free Press, 1975, pp. 219–232.

Klein, M. (1937). Love, guilt and reparation. In: R. Money-Kyrle (Ed.), *Love, Guilt and Reparation and Other Works, 1921–1945*. New York: The Free Press, 1975, pp. 306–343.

Klein, M. (1945). The Oedipus complex in light of early anxieties. In: R. Money-Kyrle (Ed.), *Love, Guilt and Reparation and Other Works, 1921–1945*. New York: The Free Press, 1975, pp. 370–419.

Klein, M. (1946). Notes on some schizoid mechanisms. In: R. Money-Kyrle (Ed.), *Envy and Gratitude and Other Works, 1946–1963*. New York: The Free Press, 1975, pp. 1–24.

Klein, M. (1959). Our adult world and its roots in infancy. In: R. Money-Kyrle (Ed.), *Envy and Gratitude and Other Works, 1946–1963*. New York: The Free Press, 1975, pp. 247–263.

Klein, G. (1976). *Psychoanalytic Theory*. New York: International Universities Press.

Kohut, H. (1959). Introspection, empathy, and psychoanalysis: An examination of the relationship between mode of observation and theory. *Journal of the American Psychoanalytic Association*. 7:459–483.

Kohut, H. (1971/2009). *The Analysis of the Self*. Chicago: University of Chicago Press.

Kohut, H. (1977). *The Restoration of the Self*. New York: International Universities Press.

Kohut, H. (1984). *How does Analysis Cure?* Chicago: University of Chicago Press.

Kohut, H., & Wolf, E. (1978). The disorders of the self and their treatment: An outline. *International Journal of Psychoanalysis*. 59:413–425.

Kris, E. (1936). The psychology of caricature. *International Journal of Psychoanalysis*. 17:285–303.

Lament, C. (2013). Three contextual frameworks for siblingships: Nonlinear thinking, disposition, and phallocentrism. *Psychoanalytic Study of the Child*. 67:84–99.

Laplanche, J., & Pontalis, J.B. (1973). *The Language of Psychoanalysis*, trans. Nicolson-Smith. London: The Hogarth Press.
Lear, J. (1998). *Love and its Place in Nature: A Philosophical Interpretation of Freudian Psychoanalysis*. New Haven, CT: Yale University Press.
Levenson, D. (1978). *The seasons of a man's life*. New York: Knopf.
Levenson, E. (1972). *The Fallacy of Understanding*. New York: Basic Books.
Litowitz, B.E. (2007). Unconscious fantasy: A once and future concept. *Journal of the American Psychoanalytic Association*. 55:199–228.
Loewald, H. (1981). Regression: Some general considerations. *Psychoanalytic Quarterly*. 50:22–43.
Lombardi, R. (2007). Shame in relation to the body, sex, and death: A clinical exploration of the psychotic levels of shame. *Psychoanalytic Dialogues*, 17:385–399.
Macalpine, I. (1950). The development of the transference. *Psychoanalytic Quarterly*. 19:501–539.
Mahler, M. (1975). *The Psychological Birth of the Human Infant*. New York: Basic Books.
Masson, J., trans., and ed. (1985). *The Complete Letters of Sigmund Freud to Wilhelm Fliess*. Cambridge, MA: Harvard University Press.
Mayes, L.C. (2001). The twin poles of order and chaos: Development as a dynamic, self-ordering system. *Psychoanalytic Study of the Child*. 56:137–170.
Mitchell, J. (2013). Siblings: Thinking theory. *Psychoanalytic Study of the Child*. 67:14–34.
Mitchell, S.A. (1988). *Relational Concepts in Psychoanalysis: An Integration*. Cambridge, MA: Harvard University Press.
Mitchell, S.A., & Greenberg, J.R. (1983). *Object Relations in Psychoanalytic Theory*. Cambridge, MA: Harvard University Press.
Modell, A. (1990). *Other Times, Other Realities: Toward a Theory of Psychoanalytic Treatment*. Cambridge, MA: Harvard University Press.
Modell, A. (1991). The therapeutic relationship as a paradoxical experience. *Psychoanalytic Dialogues*. 1:13–28.
Monsour, A. (1985). *The Structure and Dynamics of the Adolescent Self-Concept*. Unpublished doctoral dissertation, University of Denver.
Nelson, K. (1996). *Language in Cognitive Development*. Cambridge: Cambridge University Press.
Ogden, T. (1982). *Projective Identification and Psychotherapeutic Technique*. New York: Aronson.
Ogden, T. (2009). *Rediscovering Psychoanalysis: Thinking and Dreaming, Learning and Forgetting*. The New Library of Psychoanalysis Series. London, UK: Routledge.
Panksepp, J. (1998). *Affective Neuroscience: The Foundations of Human and Animal Emotions*. New York: Oxford University Press.
Popper, K. (1935/2002). *The Logic of Scientific Discovery*. New York: Routledge.
Racker, H. (1968/1982). *Transference and Countertransference*. London: Karnac.
Rangell, L. (1981). Psychoanalysis and dynamic psychotherapy—Similarities and differences twenty-five years later. *The Psychoanalytic Quarterly*. 50:665–693.
Ricoeur, P. (2012). *On Psychoanalysis*. Cambridge, U.K.: Polity Press.
Rizzolo, G.S. (2012). Rethinking Tavistock: Enactment, the Analytic Third, and the Implications for Group Relations. *Psychoanalytic Psychology*, 29:346–367.
Rizzolo, G.S. (2014). The intrapsychic and interactional realms: A hermeneutic approach to mental space. *Journal of the American Psychoanalytic Association*. 62:423–453.

Rizzolo, G.S. (2016). The critique of regression: The person, the field and the lifespan. *Journal of the American Psychoanalytic Association*. 64:1097–1031.

Rizzolo, G.S. (2017). The specter of the primitive. *The Journal of the American Psychoanalytic Association*. 65:945–977.

Rizzolo, G.S. (in press). *The Life Cycle* (without regression). *The Psychoanalytic Study of the Child*.

Robertson Smith, W. (1894/1974). *Lectures on the Religion of the Semites*, T.O. Beidelman (Ed.). Chicago: University of Chicago Press.

Rosch, E., & Lloyd, B., eds. (1978). *Cognition and Categorization*. Hillsdale, NJ: Erlbaum.

Rosenberg, M. (1979). *Conceiving the Self*. New York: Basic Books.

Sandler, J., & Freud, A. (1983). Discussions in the Hampstead Index of *The Ego and the Mechanisms of Defense*. *Journal of the American Psychoanalytic Association*, 31(Suppl.):9–146.

Sandler, J., & Sandler, A. (1984). The past unconscious, the present unconscious, and interpretation of transference. *Psychoanalytic Inquiry*. 4:367–399.

Sandler, J., & Sandler, A. (1987). The past unconscious, the present unconscious and the vicissitudes of guilt. *International Journal of Psychoanalysis*. 68:331–341.

Sandler, J., & Sandler, A. (1994a). The past unconscious and the present unconscious: A contribution to a technical frame of reference. *Psychoanalytic Study of the Child*. 49:278–292.

Sandler, J., & Sandler, A. (1994b). Regression and anti-regression. *Canadian Journal of Psychoanalysis*. 2:119–132.

Santoro, J. (1997). *The Angry Heart: Overcoming Borderline and Addictive Disorders*. Oakland, CA: New Harbinger Publications.

Sarnoff, C. (1976). *Latency*. New York: Jason Aronson.

Schafer, R. (1976). *A New Language for Psychoanalysis*. New Haven, CT: Yale University Press.

Schafer, R. (1982). The relevance of the 'here and now' transference interpretation to the reconstruction of early development. *The International Journal of Psychoanalysis*, 63:77–82.

Schliermacher, F. (1838). *Hermeneutics and Criticism and Other Writings*, trans. A. Bowie. Cambridge: Cambridge University Press, 1998.

Segal, H. (1989). Preface. In: M. Feldman & E.B. Spillius (Eds.), *Psychic Equilibrium and Psychic Change: Selected Papers of Betty Joseph*. New York: Routlege, 1989, pp. vii–ix.

Selman, R.L., & Shultz, L.H. (1990). *Making a Friend in Youth: Developmental Theory and Pair Therapy*. Chicago: University of Chicago Press.

Shengold, L. (1985). Defensive anality and anal narcissism. *International Journal of Psychoanalysis*. 66:47–73.

Sherrod, L.R. (1981). Issues in cognitive-perceptual development: The special case of social stimuli. In: M.E. Lamb & L.R. Sherrod (Eds.), *Infant Social Cognition*. Hillsdale, NJ: Erlbaum.

Solms, M., & Turnbull, O. (2002). *The Brain and the Inner World*. New York: Other Press.

Spence, D.P. (1982). *Narrative Truth and Historical Truth: Meaning and Interpretation in Psychoanalysis*. New York: W. W. Norton & Company.

Spencer, H. (1898). The Principles of Sociology. Vol. 1. New York: Appleton.

Spillius, E.B. (1999). Introduction. In: A. Ferro (Ed.), *The Bi-Personal Field. Ferro*. New York: Routledge.

Sterba, R. (1934). The fate of the ego in analytic therapy. *International Journal of Psychoanalysis*. 15:117–126.

Stern, D.B. (1983). Unformulated experience: From familiar chaos to creative disorder. *Contemporary Psychoanalysis*. 19:71–99.

Stern, D.B. (1985). *The Interpersonal World of the Infant: A View from Psychoanalysis and Developmental Psychology*. New York: Basic Books.

Stern, D.B. (2003a). The fusion of horizons: Dissociation, enactment, and understanding. *Psychoanalytic Dialogues*. 13:843–873.

Stern, D.B. (2003b). *Unformulated Experience: From Dissociation to Imagination in Psychoanalysis*. New York: Routledge.

Stern, D.B. (2005). Introduction. In: Edgar A. Levenson (Ed.), *The Fallacy of Understanding and the Ambiguity of Change*. New York: Routledge.

Stern, D.B. (2010). *Partners in Thought: Working with Unformulated Experience, Dissociation, and Enactment*. New York: Routledge.

Stern, D.B. (2015). *Relational Freedom: Emergent Properties of the Interpersonal Field*. New York: Routledge.

Stern, S. (1994). Needed relationships and repeated relationships: An integrated relational perspective. *Psychoanalytic Dialogues*, 4:317–349.

Stolorow, R.D., & Atwood, G.E. (1984/2014). *Structures of Subjectivity: Explorations in Psychoanalytic Phenomenology*. New York: Routledge.

Stolorow, R.D., & Atwood, G.E. (1997). Deconstructing the myth of the neutral analyst: An alternative from intersubjective systems theory. *The Psychoanalytic Quarterly*. 66:431–449.

Stolorow, R.D., Atwood, G.E., & Brandchaft, B. (1992). Three realms of the unconscious and their therapeutic transformation. *The Psychoanalytic Review*. 79:25–30.

Stolorow, R.D., Brandchaft, B., & Atwood, G.E. (1987). *Psychoanalytic Treatment: An Intersubjective Approach*. Hillsdale, NJ: The Analytic Press.

Stolorow, R.D., Orange, D.M., & Atwood, G.E. (1998). Projective identification begone!: Commentary on paper by Susan H. Sands. *Psychoanalytic Dialogues*, 8:719–725.

Stolorow, R.D., Orange, D.M., & Atwood, G.E. (2001). Cartesian and post-Cartesian trends in relational psychoanalysis. *Psychoanalytic Psychology*, 18:468–484.

Strachey, J. (1934). The nature of the therapeutic action of psychoanalysis. *International Journal of Psychoanalysis*. 15:127–159.

Sullivan, H.S. (1940). *Conceptions of Modern Psychiatry*. Whitefish, MT: Kessinger Publishing.

Sullivan, H.S. (1953/1997). *The Interpersonal Theory of Psychiatry*. New York: W. W. Norton & Company.

Terman, D.M. (1984). The self and the Oedipus complex. *The Annual of Psychoanalysis*. 12:87–104.

Thelen, E. (2005). Dynamic systems theory and the complexity of change. *Psychoanalytic Dialogues*. 15:255–283.

Tylor, E.B. (1871). *Primitive Culture: Researches into the Development of Mythology, Philosophy, Religion, Art, and Custom*. Cambridge: Cambridge University Press.

von Baer, K.E. (1828). *Entwicklungsgeschichte der Thiere: Beobachtung und Reflexion*. Königsberg: Bornträger.

Wachtel, P.H. (2008). *Relational Theory and the Practice of Psychotherapy*. New York: The Guilford Press.

Wachtel, P.L. (2003). The surface and the depths: The metaphor of depth in psychoanalysis and the ways in which it can mislead. *Contemporary Psychoanalysis*. 39:5–26.

Waddell, M. (1998). *Inside Lives: Psychoanalysis and the Growth of the Personality*. New York: Karnac.

Westen, D. (1989). Are "primitive" object relations really preOedipal? *American Journal of Orthopsychiatry*. 59(3):331–345.

Winnicott, D.W. (1954a). Metapsychological and clinical aspects of regression within the psycho-analytical set-up. In: M. Masud R. Khan (Ed.), *Through Paediatrics to Psychoanalysis: Collected Papers*. New York: Brunner-Routledge, 1992, pp. 278–294.

Winnicott, D.W. (1954b). Withdrawal and regression. In: M. Masud R. Khan (Ed.), *Through Paediatrics to Psychoanalysis: Collected Papers*. New York: Brunner-Routledge, 1992, pp. 295–299.

Winnicott, D.W. (1955). Clinical varieties of transference. In: M. Masud R. Khan (Ed.), *Through Paediatrics to Psychoanalysis: Collected Papers*. New York: Brunner-Routledge, 1992, pp. 255–261.

Winnicott, D.W. (1965). *The Maturational Processes and the Facilitating Environment: Studies in the Theory of Emotional Development*. London: The Hogarth Press.

Wolf, E. (1988). *Treating the Self: Elements of Clinical Self Psychology*. New York: The Guilford Press.

Zetzel, E.R. (1956). Current concepts of transference. *International Journal of Psychoanalysis*. 37:369–375.

Zetzel, E.R. (1968). The so-called good hysteric. *International Journal of Psychoanalysis*. 49:256–260.

Index

For Product Safety Concerns and Information please contact our EU representative GPSR@taylorandfrancis.com
Taylor & Francis Verlag GmbH, Kaufingerstraße 24, 80331 München, Germany

www.ingramcontent.com/pod-product-compliance
Ingram Content Group UK Ltd.
Pitfield, Milton Keynes, MK11 3LW, UK
UKHW022026061126
477531UK00002B/59
9781138624399